Sometimes I gulp down my food so fast that I forget I've eaten. Is this dangerous?

Why can't I control my promiscuous desire to sleep with people, even strangers?

Why do I feel the need to roll on dead fish, fox droppings and anything else people find repulsive?

Why do I love my female human but hate her husband?

ABOUT THE AUTHOR

Bruce Fogle DVM, MRCVS is a practising vet, and lectures on animal behaviour at veterinary colleges internationally. He is a columnist for the *Daily Telegraph* and has written several books on the behavioural problems of pets, including *The Dog's Mind* and *The Cat's Mind*. Signet also publish a companion book, *101 Questions Your Cat Would Ask Its Vet – If Your Cat Could Talk*.

BRUCE FOGLE DVM, MRCVS

101 QUESTIONS YOUR DOG WOULD ASK ITS VET
(IF YOUR DOG COULD TALK)

ILLUSTRATED BY LALLA WARD

A SIGNET BOOK

SIGNET

Published by the Penguin Group
Penguin Books Ltd, 27 Wrights Lane, London W8 5TZ, England
Penguin Books USA Inc., 375 Hudson Street, New York, New York 10014, USA
Penguin Books Australia Ltd, Ringwood, Victoria, Australia
Penguin Books Canada Ltd, 10 Alcorn Avenue, Toronto, Ontario,
Canada M4V 3B2
Penguin Books (NZ) Ltd, 182–190 Wairau Road, Auckland 10, New Zealand

Penguin Books Ltd, Registered Offices: Harmondsworth, Middlesex, England

First published by Michael Joseph 1993
Published in Signet 1994
1 3 5 7 9 10 8 6 4 2

Printed in England by Clays Ltd, St Ives plc

Contents

Acknowledgements

The more time I spend with them – and, professionally speaking, it is now well over twenty years – the more I like dogs. I respect them, but also they make me laugh. And so, first of all, my apologies to any dogs or their people who might think, after reading some of these questions, that I'm not taking them seriously. I hope you'll see from the answers that I am. And second, my thanks and acknowledgement to the thousands of dog owners who, over the years, have asked the questions that follow. Thanks, too, to the dogs.

Introduction

In my house I used to ask simple questions, such as 'Who'd like to take the dogs for a walk to the park?' I soon stopped, because even when they were pretending to be asleep my dogs were secretly eavesdropping on human conversations. I switched to spelling – P-A-R-K, W-A-L-K – and learned that any intelligent canine knows how to spell too. I tried euphemisms. I'd ask the kids, 'Who wants to take the quadrupeds for exercise to the green place?', and instantly two wide-eyed, innocent-looking retrievers would be sitting at my feet silently saying, 'We'll take the kids.' Uncanny!

Dogs read clocks too. Mine get fed around 6.30 each evening, but if I forget, at 6.31 they sit themselves down in front of me, use secret laser vision to get my attention, and when they catch my eye, get up, go to the kitchen, walk back, and silently but explicitly ask me to follow. I know a cocker spaniel who speaks even more directly. When she is hungry, she picks up her food bowl, carries it to her human and drops it at his feet.

Most impressive of all are multilingual dogs, especially those that understand conditional statements in different languages. At only a few months of age, these brilliant linguists know what is meant when either their non-English-speaking owners or I say, 'If you do that once more I'll be really angry.'

OK, I exaggerate. Dogs can't spell, read clocks or understand conditional clauses. They understand a good but limited range of human sounds and soon learn that when they hear 'walk' or 'marche' something exciting follows. They have superb twenty-four-hour biological clocks that help them to remember the timing of important events like feeding time. They understand people's moods through voice inflection rather than the word content of their speech.

I don't think I'm alone in enjoying the 'human-ness' of dogs, in liking to think they *really* understand. If I issue a command to my cat, she makes a rude gesture with a forepaw and saunters off. I need only whisper my dogs' names and they are at my feet, looking up into my eyes, telling me I'm the most important person in the whole world – not bad for the ego. When there is a noise outside my house and my dogs bark and run to the window or door, I enjoy the feeling that they will protect me. When I come home in the evening and they greet me as if I have just come back from the voyage in *The Odyssey*, they give me a feeling of fidelity that few human relations can provide. And when they settle down to be stroked and I settle down too, stroking them, it is curiously reassuring that in a changing world there is also permanence, certainty, constancy.

For a variety of reasons we communicate better with dogs than with any other domesticated species. We understand them because we share a surprisingly wide variety of behaviours with them. That is why the dog was the first animal we domesticated and why he is both proverbially and literally 'man's best friend'.

A teacher once asked this question of her twelve-year-old students: 'You see your dog and a man you have never met before fall in the river. Which one will you save first?' Most of her pupils would rescue their pet first. Their replies exemplify the fact that in both North American and northern European cultures the dog is considered to be part of the family, with rights and privileges of other family members. By accepting dogs as individuals with distinctive personalities (and sometimes even endowing them with human characteristics), it helps us to understand their needs and afflictions, and reinforces the obligations we have towards them as pets.

That is one reason why dogs are asking the questions in this book. I want to reinforce the fact that if we keep them as companions, we have obligations to understand them, care for them and make their lives actively pleasant, although we don't always have to rescue them first. A second reason for putting these questions in canine mouths is that I don't think it is such a terribly bad thing to humanise dogs a little. It reminds us that they can feel jealousy, act petulant, experience elation and suffer sadness.

What I hope you will also understand is that they are *not* human. They share their behaviours with the wolf. All we have done through domestication is to diminish some wolf characteristics and enhance others. As much a part of the family as they are, pet dogs always remain wolves in disguise. They carry a veneer of human culture, but in the absence of human control, they can revert to their natural behaviour.

The following questions might be asked by most

dogs. However, because of the dog's limited attention span and easy boredom threshold, the answers were written with both canines and their human families in mind, for in the end, it is the humans who will find the answers most useful.

If your dog has a question, no matter how trivial you may think it is, please send it to me:

Bruce Fogle
Dog Questions
c/o Michael Joseph Ltd
27 Wrights Lane
London W8 5TZ

I'll try to include it in future editions.

CHAPTER ONE

Instincts and Communication

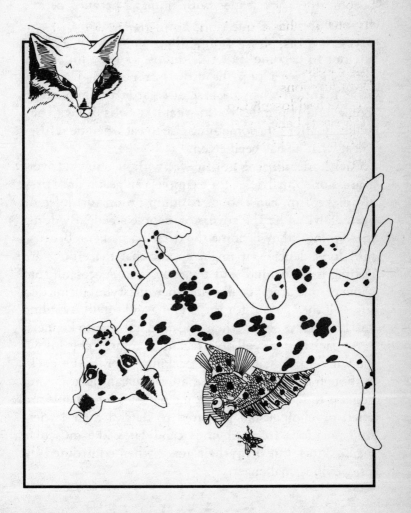

1. I want to be the pack leader with people. How should I go about it?

Disobey. Even the puniest, most insignificant dog can become the pack leader with humans because people are such pushovers.

People often don't notice the first signs of a dog's attempt to become leader of the pack. They think it is cute when, as a pup, he growls at people. They pay little attention when he first disregards a command to 'come' and continues to do whatever he is doing. They willingly offer him something else to eat when he refuses to eat what he has been given.

Pack leadership can be achieved without showing overt aggression. Small dogs, for example, can pester until they are picked up, can choose to jump up on furniture or even crawl under the covers on people's beds. By doing these things, they become the decision makers. Because they look delicate, it might appear that these dogs are leading from behind, but the ploy is so successful that some people dramatically alter their lifestyles, hiring dog sitters if they go out for the evening and totally avoiding yearly holidays so that their dog need not go into kennels.

As pack animals, all dogs feel most comfortable knowing where they stand in the pecking order of the pack. Although sex, size and breed are significant factors, any dog has the potential to become pack leader. People are often psychologically prepared to defend their leadership positions from obvious candidates like muscular male Akitas, but drop their guard when confronted by less obvious challengers.

2. I have an overwhelming need to sniff trees and stick my nose almost right into other dogs' droppings. And I can't help sticking my snout in the crutches of unfamiliar humans. Am I a pervert?

Reading smells is like reading newspapers, only better. Scents pass on today's news. By sniffing another dog's body waste products, a canine can tell the sex of the depositor, how recently that other dog has passed, if he is a male how 'masculine' he is, and if a female, whether she is coming into season or is already there. He might even be able to determine his or her emotional state.

After a dog empties his bowels, he anoints the deposit with two drops from his anal sacs, special scent-marking glands on either side of the anus. Anal sac secretions contain dozens of different odour-producing chemicals; each one probably contains specific information for the sniffer. Similarly plain urine has very little odour, but hormones make it smell quite distinctive and pass on a wealth of information about the sexual and emotional status of the producer. These odours are not smelled in the nose: dogs have a special sex-sniffing apparatus, the vomeronasal organ, which humans don't have. They investigate new humans by inhaling crutch odours into this apparatus. Curiously, dogs only crutch-sniff strange humans, but arm- and leg-sniff ones they know, in each instance searching out specific odour information. Humans find it difficult to comprehend how superbly dogs communicate using body odours simply because they have comparatively primitive abilities.

3. Why do I kick dirt after emptying my bowels or bladder?

Dogs don't need to be trained to kick dirt. It is a basic instinct. However, some dogs who don't kick dirt can learn to do so by watching other dogs. When they are quite young, pups have the ability to watch and learn how to kick dirt, but this inclination to copy generally is lost as they grow older.

Body waste products are good substances for marking territories, so rather than simply dropping them randomly, dogs will use them to leave messages. The discharges themselves are quite innocuous, however, so some dogs highlight them by kicking up earth beside or even on top of them. This has two purposes: it makes the site more visibly obvious, and it releases ground scents that another passing dog might pick up. Once these smells are noticed, it is more likely that the urine or faeces will be noted too.

Males are more likely to kick dirt than females simply because they have a greater urge to mark territory, although females kick more after they have been spayed. Kicking is completely different from digging, because the hind legs are used randomly to kick backwards; digging involves a rather studious and concentrated use of the forepaws.

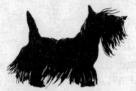

4. Why do I compulsively feel the need to roll on dead fish, fox droppings and anything else that people find repulsive?

Just as many people enjoy masking their personal body odours with artificial ones, so do dogs. Dogs find certain odours appealing, and usually prefer the smell of decomposing organic material, such as leaf mould, rotting fish and fertiliser.

Applying canine perfume is almost always performed in a ritual manner. If a dog simply wants to have a playful role, he will quite carelessly throw himself on his back – sometimes even somersaulting to do so – and, arching left and right, kick his legs up in the air. He then gets up and trots along.

When applying perfume, however, a dog is much more particular. He carefully sniffs his chosen cologne. If it is 'bottled' like a dead fish, he might carry it from the beach onto grass and lay it out in an exact manner. Then quite studiously, like a human applying perfume behind one ear and then the other, he rubs on his substance with one shoulder and then the other. At this stage he might not even roll. Instead he inhales the perfume once more and, reinvigorated by the aroma, applies the substance once more to his shoulders and then, using a full roll, to his back. This is a clever move for an animal that in the wild must stalk and kill other animals in order to survive. If he masks his own odour and is up-wind to a potential meal, that meal will probably not be too concerned if it thinks it is being approached by a dead fish.

5. *Sometimes I get so excited when people come home that I wet myself. How can I learn to control my bladder?*

Dogs who wet themselves when they greet people lack self-esteem. To stop doing it they need to gain confidence.

People should always be at the top of the totem pole in the dog pack hierarchy. All dogs should demonstrate submissiveness when their people come home, but a simple wag of the tail is all that is really needed. More overt displays of fealty to human leaders – whining, grovelling, rolling over or, worst, rolling over and urinating – are unnecessary.

Often unwittingly people reassert their leadership by reaching down from their considerable height and patting the dog on the top of the head. If people act this way with an insecure dog, she wets herself. To correct the problem people should avoid touching the insecure dog immediately; instead, they should come in the house without making eye contact. After a few minutes they should stoop to reduce their height and, still avoiding eye contact, put forward an upturned palm and let the dog make the decision to come forward. When she does come forward, the person tickles her under the chin but still doesn't look at her or speak to her. Perfectly natural human greeting rituals, such as eye contact and verbal 'hellos', are gestures of dominance to dogs. If people avoid using them, the insecure dog has a chance to improve her self-worth. When she does that, she learns to control her bladder too.

6. Why do I feel the need to bark so loudly when strangers approach the house? Humans have threatened me with debarking.

Any sensible dog considers himself to be a member of a pack and his house to be the most important part of his pack's territory. Although the role of pack leader always goes to humans, all members of the pack are equally responsible for warning others when their territory is about to be invaded. And the best way to warn all others instantly is to bark.

For thousands of years humans have interfered in dog breeding, turning the comparatively quiet wolf into the yapping dog. Because a dog's hearing is about four times more acute than a human's, dogs make good guards. Now, after intentionally selecting for and enhancing barking, humans have decided that it is a dog trait they don't particularly want.

Some breeds bark more than others. Generally speaking, small dogs, especially terriers, are yappers, while large dogs, especially gun dogs, are relatively quiet. Debarking is an operation in which holes are punched in the dog's vocal cords. Except in Japan, where barking is a dog's most heinous crime, very few veterinarians are ever willing to carry out the operation. Instead vets suggest finding out why the dog feels the need to bark and then retraining him accordingly. When this proves impossible, they might try a curious bark-stopping method developed in France that involves the dog wearing a special collar containing a vial of citronella. When the dog barks, a microchip in the collar is activated and the lemon scent of citronella envelops the barker. This innocuous smell acts as an instant distraction. In a short period of time many dogs will not bark whenever they are wearing their personal odour-maker.

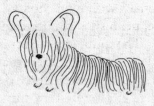

7. Why do I howl when I hear Beethoven?

Howling is a form of communication. Dogs howl to tell each other where they are. Whether they are trying to communicate with Beethoven when they howl is questionable, however.

Wolves use the prototypical howl to speak to each other. When, for example, a pack is dispersed in the woods and a lonely wolf pup yips a 'Where is everybody?' yip, eerie, primitive, plaintive and quite beautiful howls respond. The pup stops yipping. Young dogs also yip when left alone. As they mature some dogs, especially hounds and Dobermanns, develop mournful howls. When they are lonely they turn their heads skywards, purse their lips and bay.

Loneliness is not the only reason for howling. Some dogs howl when greeting people. Others howl when they are happy, and some howl to music. A dog's hearing range is about the same as a human's, roughly eight and a half octaves, but their sensitivity within that range is quite acute. They can, for example, differentiate between two notes differing by only one-eighth of a tone. This explains why dogs learn to respond to a shepherd's whistled commands so easily.

Deep in one of the most basic parts of their brains humans have a music centre. Dogs probably do too. Music is relaxing. It can be calming and reassuring to animals. Howling to Beethoven – or to any other music for that matter – is always actively performed by the howler: a dog joins in because he wants to. It's enjoyable. If the sound of music were unpleasant, he would simply get up and leave.

8. Humans smile a lot. Can I learn how to do it too?

Dogs don't naturally smile with happiness. Smiling is a behaviour of primates. Chimpanzees smile. So do orangutans. These primates kiss on the lips too, just like their fellow primates, humans, do, and this is often associated with happy smiling. Although dogs like licking other dogs' lips or even a human's lips, it's not exactly the same. Lip-licking does mean friendship, but in a non-sexual context it usually denotes subservience. Retracting the lips into what to humans looks like a smile is really a sign of submission. Visiting the veterinarian, for example – no laughing matter to most dogs – causes many to retract their lips, but at the same time they cower behind their human's legs and shiver.

Some dogs do smile when they are happy and have learned to do it by mimicking humans. Potentially any dog can learn to smile, but terriers seem to be the best students. They must start by watching people smile while they are still puppies. Rather than retracting the lips in a smile-like grin, a smile-mimicker raises his upper lips and shows his teeth. Showing off his weapons is normally a sign of aggression, but when it is performed as a smile the lips retract at the same time. Unfortunately, dogs are simply not made to smile, so when the upper lip raises, the nose wrinkles and this almost invariably results in a sneeze. Aggressive weapon displays are accompanied by growls; smiling weapon displays are accompanied by tail wags and silly snorts.

9. I live with a cat and enjoy her company, so why do I always feel this urge to chase any other cat I see?

Dogs instinctively chase anything that moves fast, especially if it is small and furry, but when personal relationships develop they usually draw the line. When a dog and cat live together, the cat usually dominates. If a dog becomes too nosey or inquisitive, a confident cat hisses, spits and swipes her canine companion into line. In good, stable relationships, the cat will sleep contentedly with the dog, eat in the same room at the same time, and use a wagging tail as a plaything and the dog's forelimbs as scratching posts. Dogs are usually fascinated by cats and allow them to do all these things.

Strange cats are treated differently. When there are no formal relationships, dogs chase cats just as dogs chase squirrels. This is an instinctive reaction at the very base of dog behaviour and is independent of sex, age or hunger. Rapid movement stimulates the chase. This can put a pet at risk, especially if she lives with two or more canines. Even when dogs are on perfectly amicable terms with a cat, the dogs can go native and chase their friend if they see her run. This is less likely to happen in a single dog household.

Chasing is a good game, but the great risk comes from the fact that it is self-perpetuating. Chasing stimulates a rush of adrenalin. Dogs find that invigorating, so when they are offered the opportunity, they will chase again. The more often they chase, the more likely they are to catch a cat, and possibly even to kill it.

10. People think I'm primitive and want to move me out of the house just because they are bringing home a baby. Is this fair?

If a dog already lives in the house, it is usually totally unnecessary and possibly even counter-productive to move him outdoors when a baby is brought home.

Once more, the dog's response to a new baby is conditioned by his need to know his place in the pack. Dogs don't like change. They feel most secure when life is full of satisfying routines. New human babies will upset these routines, so people should plan the home-coming in advance by gradually altering routines while they still have the energy to do so.

If a dog has been treated as a child substitute, lavished with time and affection, played with, spoken to, petted, cuddled and fawned over, these treatments should become gradually more sporadic. Rather than letting the dog initiate feeding, exercise or affection, humans should become the initiators. If he must learn to sleep in a new place, now is the time that he should move. This will diminish the dog's feeling of superiority. When the baby is brought home, the dog can be 'rewarded' by letting him smell all the new smells. At this point no other routines should be changed. As long as the dog continues to receive the attention he deserves, he won't feel anything other than a little sibling rivalry. After several months, once he discovers that human infants are not as tidy with their food as dog infants, that they drop or even throw it on the floor, he will positively come to enjoy the presence of the new baby.

11. I enjoyed watching television when I lived in Europe, but now that I have moved to America all I see is a blur. What has happened to my eyes?

Television is better for dogs to watch in Europe than in North America. Aside from the fact that in Europe dogs are more likely than those in North America to see sheepdog trials, show jumping and natural history shows – all favourite programmes – differences in transmission quality mean that dogs see TV pictures in Europe but only dots in America.

Until high-definition television becomes readily available, American dogs are restricted to watching an inferior system that transmits pictures so slowly all they see are dots on the screen. If these unfortunate canines hear Lassie, Benji or Rin Tin Tin barking, they look behind the television to see where the dog is.

European dogs have no difficulty seeing television images because both kinds of European TV transmission system are faster than the American one, fast enough to form images that dogs can see. This means that if there is a good programme on TV, the European dog will settle down and watch it. People need not invest in colour TV, however. Although dogs have cells in their eyes and in their brains that can form colour images, they are completely uninterested in colour and are happy to see in shades of grey.

12. Why do I dig so many holes in the ground and then just leave them?

Digging is both mentally and physically stimulating. This form of open-face mining is a dead-end behaviour in many dogs. They do it because it is an instinctive behaviour that once served a useful purpose.

Although wolves classically feast on large herbivores, such as deer, they also eat a surprisingly large number of small rodents. Wolves use a cat-like pounce to capture wandering rodents. However, rather than sit patiently at a den as a cat will when she is waiting for her meal to emerge, the typical wolf uses his forepaws to dig where the rodent has gone to ground until he finds his prey. This is one reason why dogs dig holes and leave them.

Because in the wild there are times when food is plentiful and other times when food is scarce, wolves often cache excess food. When stomachs have been filled, they dig in the earth and bury parts of carcasses for future consumption. Dogs do this with bones, of course, but today few dogs are given bones to chew. The desire to cache food remains, so on a full stomach a dog might dig a hole but, having nothing to drop in it, will simply leave it.

Dogs also dig out of boredom, or to escape, but in the end they do it because it stimulates the senses. As well as refreshing the muscles, digging releases a cornucopia of smells from the ground, many of which are organic in origin and lip-smackingly good. Worms, bugs, decomposing matter, moisture: all of these are a delight to the inquisitive canine's senses.

13. *Although I am a physically mature male, I am embarrassed that I don't know how to cock my leg. Should I be concerned?*

The only concern for a male dog who does not cock his leg is that he shoots himself each time he urinates. Leg-cocking is stimulated by scent, by hormones and by observation. If, for example, a female puppy is raised *only* with male dogs and only smells male urine, she might learn to cock her leg a little when she urinates, even though there is no anatomical reason to do so. If she is spayed before she reaches puberty, she will continue to cock her leg.

Dogs cock their legs to leave urine scent at the nose level of other dogs. These scent marks are left throughout the dog's territory as reminders of who owns it. All pups start out life by squatting to urinate, but even as young pups some males will cock their legs. That is because they have already produced some male hormone, testosterone, even before they were born and this hormone has made their brains 'masculine'. Another result of this masculinisation is that these pups might mount and thrust on other pups in spite of the fact that they are only weeks old and months away from puberty.

At the other extreme, even after reaching puberty some dogs still go on squatting to urinate. They have normal levels of circulating male hormone. They have viable sperm and are as fertile as other males, but take longer or don't develop the male habit of leg-lifting. There is no harm in this, but if a dog wants to learn to lift his leg he should spend time with leg-cocking males.

14. I've been told that sometimes when I am asleep my face twitches and my legs flail in the air. Apparently I cry or howl. What's happening?

Dogs dream more vividly than most humans. They rest frequently during the day, often falling into a light but alert sleep from which they instantly emerge when any of their senses are stimulated. Bored dogs will sleep more deeply during the day and, just as they do at night, will experience periods of deep sleep during which they dream.

As pack members, dogs co-ordinate their activities with their humans. Because humans enjoy prolonged night-time sleeping, most dogs do the same, although if given their preference they would prefer to be up at the crack of dawn. As dogs go from light sleep to deep sleep their eyes start to move under their closed lids. This happens to people too. Electrical changes occur in the brains of both dogs and humans; while most people dream quietly, dogs dream more robustly. First their whiskers twitch, then their lips move and sometimes their jaws chew and their tongues lick. At the same time, their paw muscles retract and they start paddling with their feet, making Disneyesque running movements. Some utter short crying yips or howls. Although human dreams last about twenty minutes, dog dreams are much shorter – either the rabbit is caught or it is not. The dog then falls back into a light sleep but will dream several more times before the night is out.

15. Whenever I visit another home I enjoy urinating on the walls, especially if I can smell another dog. My people want to take me to a psychiatrist. Is that really necessary?

No, it isn't. Just as dogs scent-mark trees and shrubs, they also naturally urine-mark walls, curtains and table legs. In fact, when visiting the veterinary clinic it is not unknown for them to inhale deeply and urine-mark on the veterinarian's trousers.

People seldom behave in the same way, and find this form of canine communication offensive. Technically speaking, his behaviour is typical, so there is no need for a psychiatrist. Good counselling, however, is always welcome.

Dogs should learn that territory marking is permissible outdoors but forbidden in either their own or any other indoor environment. Training involves rewarding the dog when he enters a home and behaves according to human requirements and punishing him when he behaves 'normally'. Punishment should be psychological rather than physical. Theatrical gestures, such as suddenly raised voices, water pistols, noise makers and perfectly aimed small bean bags, might prevent the marking gesture, but if these fail people should instantly remove the dog from the scene of the misdemeanour and isolate him for a symbolic minute. This form of discipline often works, but when it doesn't, interfering with the sex hormone, testosterone, does. People can achieve this either by feeding or injecting their dog with anti-male or female hormone or by castrating him.

16. Why do I sometimes feel the urge to bite people's ankles just when they're about to leave the room?

This is a curious learned behaviour and is a simple but effective manifestation of canine bossiness. When people gather together in the presence of an ankle-biting dog, they might think that the dog is an irrelevant member of the quorum, but the dog thinks he is the supremo. He likes to think that he is the centre of activity and that people have gathered for his benefit.

He might behave perfectly normally, offering sociable greetings to everyone, chatting about the weather, asking about the kids and being generously affectionate, allowing people – even asking them – to stroke him and talk to him. A perfect host. But as they leave he undergoes a complete personality change. He has enjoyed the company and doesn't want it to end, but people are leaving without his permission. So he eats ankle.

The procedure is rewarding because it is so effective: bite a departing ankle and you not only become the centre of attention and assert your authority, but you also delay your guests from leaving. That is why dogs will do the same thing on the next visit from humans. People can prevent this form of canine dominance either by not letting the dog mix with company or, quite simply, by removing him well before their human guests depart.

CHAPTER TWO

Emotions and Behaviour

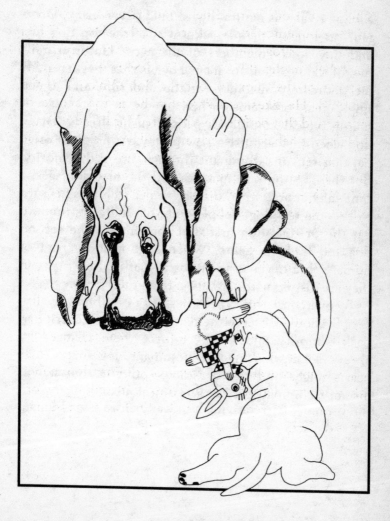

17. I know I'm loved, but I still feel jealous when I see people petting the old dog I live with. So I bit him. How can I control this selfish side of myself?

Sibling rivalry is natural but should never lead to problems as long as people acknowledge the top dog first and then lower members of the pack. Unfortunately, one of the problems humans have is that they naturally feel more responsibility for the underdog and unwittingly create problems for her.

In a typical household, people might already have a dog when they acquire a new puppy. At first, the original dog remains dominant through size and seniority. But then, as the pup matures and the first dog ages, a time might come when the newcomer feels it is his turn to become top dog. People quite naturally continue to pat the original dog first, but this annoys the second dog and leads to fights. When dogs fight in front of humans, but never in their absence, it is almost certain they are disputing for attention from their people.

To overcome this type of jealousy or sibling rivalry, people should observe the natural changes occurring in pack seniority and then reinforce these changes by always acknowledging the dominant dog first. Their hearts might find this a difficult practice, but it will instantly eliminate further acts of jealousy.

18. Why do I love my female human but hate her husband?

It could be that she smells nicer. Dogs can be jealous, and they can be protective over what they consider to be theirs. In any dog-human relationship one human in particular becomes the paramount pack leader. Leadership will vary from household to household. In some homes a dog picks her feeder and walker as her leader: this is often a female human. Yet in other homes a dog will choose as her commander-in-chief the person with the lowest, sternest voice, usually the male person. Dogs who choose these males are more likely to be innately dominant canines.

Sex and jealousy are more important factors in liking women but hating men. Dogs raised in female environments become accustomed to women's voices and odours. They feel secure in the presence of women because their behaviour, looks, movements, odours and sounds are familiar. If they are male dogs, they also become proprietorial over these human females and feel threatened when they smell men.

Dog jealousy is not an uncommon situation. Some dogs will go so far as to try to prevent a husband getting in bed with his wife. 'She's *mine!*' they say as they snap at the man's ankles. This form of canine hate can be diminished by having the man take over some rewarding responsibilities, such as feeding and playing with the dog.

19. Each time I see the new people next door I growl and threaten. There is just something about them that I don't like. My humans don't like my behaviour. How can I control it?

Some dogs are deeply suspicious of anything or anybody new. Neighbours, in particular, can be troublesome because they remain so close to a dog's territory and never go away. They are constantly threatening. If they have a dog, the threat is even more real.

This type of problem is, in fact, quite easy to overcome. All that is necessary is for the threatened dog to think that the new neighbours and their dog are simply new members of an extended pack. The dogs and neighbours should meet first on neutral territory, in the local park for example. The dog will see that these new people and their dog are no threat to his humans. The dog can be offered a little food by the neighbours, and if there are even the remotest signs of canine aggression the delinquent dog should be firmly admonished.

Once the neighbours and their dogs are able to meet in the park with no troubles, they proceed to meet on the dog's home territory, both outside and inside. It takes a very short time for a dog to accept that there is no threat intended from the new humans and only a little longer to accept that the new canine isn't a threat either.

20. I'm mean and nasty. What type of muzzle should I use?

Muzzles should allow a dog to pant freely or even to drink but should prevent her from biting. Any dog should be muzzled if she is placed in a situation where she might bite. The softest, gentlest canine might bite when she is in pain. If a dog has been injured, she should be muzzled temporarily while she is taken to the veterinary clinic.

Members of breeds that are known to be potentially snappy should always be muzzled when they first meet crawling children. Kids don't mean to hurt dogs, but it is no fun to be yanked by your hair, and a typical terrier's response is to snap at the yanker. Only when people are convinced that there are no dangers should an unmuzzled dog be allowed to be with young children and then only in the presence of adults.

Some dogs are unpredictable, and they should be muzzled whenever they are off their own territory. This means they should wear a muzzle when visiting the veterinary clinic, when exercising, when being walked and whenever they are off the lead. Some people like to put heavy studded leather muzzles on their dogs. These are unpleasant for dogs and unnecessary. Instead, dogs should wear either a basket-like muzzle that allows complete air circulation, or a nylon cone-like one that slips on the nose but allows enough space for the tongue to come out for panting or lapping. Dogs initially don't like wearing muzzles, but if they are introduced to them gently, they soon accept them and wear them with nonchalance.

21. Recently there was an upset in my life and my favourite person is no longer here. Now all I want to do is lie around looking miserable. Is this dog depression?

Yes, it is. Dogs have emotions and suffer from depression just as humans do. What dogs enjoy most is constancy. They form emotional attachments to other dogs and to people, and can be upset when these attachments are broken.

That doesn't mean that all dogs get depressed when there are major changes in their lives. Once more, just like people, some adapt better than others. Those most likely to suffer are dogs that have formed deep dependent relationships with one person or one dog in particular. In other words, followers are more likely to become depressed than leaders. The problem can be reduced by ensuring that dogs treat all human members of their pack as co-leaders, so that when one is absent there is another to whom the dog can show allegiance.

Temporary separations cause only temporary depression but permanent separation is more difficult for a dog to understand. Although the value is questionable, there is no harm in letting a surviving dog see and sniff the body of another household pet that has died recently. When people die or move away, another person should immediately take over leadership responsibilities, making sure that the dog receives affection, touch, nourishment and discipline. When this is done, depression lasts only a short time and virtually never requires medical treatment.

22. I hate being left alone, so when it happens I rampage through the house to amuse myself. But why do I also eat houseplants, chew furniture and urinate on the bed?

Dogs are gregariously sociable animals. They relish activity, not necessarily because they want to participate in it, although most do, but because just watching is mentally stimulating. Unless a dog is unwell or of a retiring disposition he wants to be in the middle of the action. When people have other people over to the house the dog wants to greet and investigate them, join them for drinks and help with the barbecue. He doesn't like being left out.

Being left alone is unnatural and boring. Dogs living with humans soon learn that when they are bored they need only search out another member of the human pack and they will be touched, talked to, played with, fed, or even admonished – this, too, is a form of attention. Attention is what most dogs want. When the entire human pack leaves the dog alone he becomes anxious, agitated and frustrated. In his anxiety he becomes destructive.

His destructive activities are not carried out in retribution for being isolated. For instance, he doesn't say to himself that he's going to urinate on the bed because he knows humans find this deeply offensive. He does things he would never do otherwise, out of anxiety and frustration. To avoid these problems, people should accustom dogs, while they are still very young pups, to be left alone. People should depart quietly, without saying 'goodbye' or making physical contact – dogs are clever at hearing hidden stress in people's voices. Two or three chewable toys should be left for the dog to play with. Leaving a radio or television on might also provide soothing background noise and help to reduce his natural anxiety to an acceptable level.

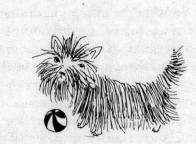

23. I am a happy and content fourteen-year-old. My people have recently decided they are going to get a puppy for me. Is this really necessary?

In most instances a new pup does wonders for an elderly dog and the family too. All dogs, even those that are firmly convinced they are human and that other dogs are aliens from outer space, ultimately enjoy canine companionship. With the exception of dogs who show senile changes or are in chronic discomfort with old age aches and pains, even dogs who have never experienced the company of another of their own kind will, within days or weeks, thank their humans for bringing into the pack something they completely understand.

An elderly dog initially does not like being leapt upon, licked, sucked, nuzzled, pummelled and chewed by a pup. He will snap at the youngster, who soon learns that the elderly deserve respect. On the other hand, pups smell delicious, they speak in much better dog language than people ever can and they act as a fountain of youth, bringing out a streak of competitiveness and playfulness in the old one.

The life expectancy of the canine old age pensioner is limited, but his death is slightly easier for people when there is another dog in the home stirring up the silent air. There is, however, a critical point in canine aging after which it is unwise for people to bring home a new pup. If an elderly dog is irreversibly mentally or physically infirm, it is best to wait until after his departure before puppifying the house.

24. Lately I've been irritable. Am I getting grumpier as I get older?

Irritability often increases with advancing age, but it frequently has a specific and treatable cause.

As life progresses, dogs become quite settled in their ways. Routine becomes more and more important, until eventually dogs will carry out specific activities, not necessarily because they want to do them but just because they have always done them. A dog might bark an 'I'm irritated' demand that he wants to go outside because he has always gone outside at that time, but once out he forgets why he wanted to go there.

With aging, a dog's senses diminish. Like humans he doesn't hear as well as he used to, and just like people he certainly can't focus his eyes as he once could. All the nerves in his body become less efficient; they don't send messages as quickly as they did. This means that sudden sights and sounds are more likely to frighten him. An unexpected touch becomes fear-inducing, and he responds with a snap of his teeth. These perfectly natural aging changes can lead to a certain grumpiness.

Irritability might also be caused by chronic low-grade discomfort. Dogs are not complainers. They simply get on with life even when they develop bone, joint and muscle weakness or pain. If it hurts when they move, they have every right to snap when people stroke them. Fortunately, this type of grumpiness frequently responds to anti-inflammatories or other appropriate medicines.

25. Thunderstorms make me panic, firecrackers make me cringe, and when I hear a car backfire I'm certain I'm dead. Why have I suddenly become so frightened by loud noises and what can I do about it?

If a dog has not been fearful of loud noises before but is now, he has learned the behaviour and it can be 'unlearned'.

Firecrackers are only set off on certain days of the year and car backfiring is infrequent and unpredictable. Thunderstorms are the noisy events that are most likely to occur frequently, and so are the events that a dog can be retrained to accept without distress or fear.

Dogs hear sounds at almost four times the distance that humans can hear them, so they know a thunderstorm is approaching before people do. They also might feel the change in ionisation in the air and associate that with their previous fear. However hard it is for them, people should not respond to the dog's fear by being protective or by trying to distract him from the sounds. These well-intentioned gestures only reinforce the fear.

Whenever possible, and this usually means a trip to a specialty record store for a sound effects tape, people should try to mimic the frightening noise, but at a much lower sound level so that it doesn't induce fear. They should not comfort the dog when he panics. However, day by day, as the sound level is increased, the dog should be rewarded for not showing fear. It usually takes about three weeks before the record of the sound can be played at real noise level with no canine response.

26. I enjoy dominating people and making life miserable for them. How long will I be able to keep it up?

Dogs can dominate people as long as people want them to, and that sometimes means for the dog's entire life. Some people are emotionally dependent on their dogs, so they make easy pushovers. Others simply don't understand dog behaviour, and before they know it they've become putty in their dog's paws.

Emotionally dependent people are the easiest to dominate. For their own personal reasons, which vary tremendously, these people make their greatest emotional investment in their dogs. In return, they allow their canine companions to become true pack leaders, to demand feeding, to be selective about what they eat, to choose when and where and with whom they sleep, to guard and protect their house from visitors and to prevent any form of unsolicited grooming.

Other dogs can get away with the same dominant activities not because their people are emotionally dependent but because they don't understand the subtleties of canine behaviour. A dog can get away with being dominant only for as long as these people remain ignorant or mystified by his behaviour. Once they understand what the dog is really doing, if they withdraw all canine privileges, if they don't allow him to get something for nothing ever again, if they command him to sit before he is fed and before he is petted, and to roll over for grooming, the humans take over pack leadership and canine dominance ends.

27. I'm well fed and well cared for, but I still hate anyone coming near my food or my toys. Is this what humans call obsessive behaviour? Can it lead to problems?

It is not an obsession. It is simply guarding behaviour, a form of jealousy. Some dogs guard their food, others their toys, and still others their people. All of these activities can lead to serious problems.

Guarding is more common in some breeds than others. It occurs with surprising frequency in golden retrievers, a breed renowned for gentleness of spirit. Male goldens in particular can be very possessive of food bowls, never allowing humans or canines near them. Many terriers act in a similar fashion, but primarily with their toys. This is a form of possessive aggression. Other variations include competition for affection from people or sibling rivalry.

Because possessiveness is a form of dog dominance and because there is a strong genetic component in the condition, prevention means selecting the right breed when you choose your pet. For example, possessiveness isn't a serious problem with pack hounds like beagles, who are bred to work together. Treating the problem means that people have to assert their authority by revealing their own dominance, especially when the dog is still young. All human members of the family must take part in commanding the dog to obey instructions such as 'sit' and 'stay'. By reducing the dog's self-confidence, people reassert their authority over him and he will become less authoritarian about his possessions.

28. I enjoy meeting people. In fact, I think they are a marvellous species. But why is it that I can't seem to get on with my own kind?

People often get dogs when the pups are around eight weeks old and then incarcerate them in dog-free environments for the following month, during which the canines are inoculated against infectious diseases. Unfortunately this is one of the most important months in the dog's entire life, for it is during this time that he acquires important knowledge about the world around him.

Between eight and twelve weeks of age a dog learns the basic social graces. Most importantly, he learns the right and wrong ways to meet other dogs. If, for example, he stays with his mother and irritates her, she bites him in a forceful yet inhibited way and he learns that there are limits to boisterousness. But in the absence of dog-to-dog encounters during this critical socialising period, he is likely to forget what he learned with his litter and instead learns how to behave socially only with humans. All sensible dogs must learn about human culture, but at the same time they need to know as much as possible about how to behave with other dogs if they are ever to enjoy dog company. This means that even before they are fully vaccinated, pups should continue to meet other healthy dogs. If this is done, the pup will mature into an adult equally at ease with humans and other canines.

29. Why do members of my own sex antagonise me and make me so angry, while members of the opposite sex not only don't bother me, but also make rather good play partners?

Members of the same sex are more likely to be competitive with each other because they are more similar than members of the opposite sex. All dogs want to know where they stand in the pack. If two dogs are the same sex, especially if they are the same age and the same breed as well, they will find it difficult to work out their ranks. A common consequence is that they fight. Theatricals don't work. They might try intimidating each other, but because they are so equal neither backs down when threatened. Even when they fight, often there is no clear winner, so they fight again.

This doesn't happen only with males. Two females of equal age, size and breed are just as likely to fight over seniority of rank time and again and fail consistently to create a firm pecking order simply because they are too equal.

When males meet females, however, there are already obvious differences between them: they smell different, look different and act different. Even if they are the same age and breed, there will often be a size difference too. All of these are ranking factors. Add to them a little ritual display, like the male making eye contact and the female avoiding his gaze, and, introductions over, rank decided, they can amble off and play like two happy dogs.

CHAPTER THREE

Training

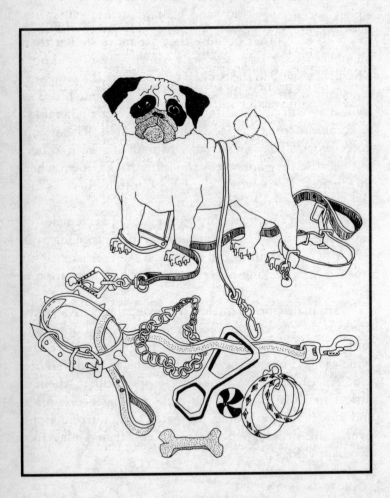

30. What forms of discipline might people use to train me and how can I best resist?

Rewards and discipline are used equally in dog training. Food and physical contact are the most potent rewards, while social isolation and harsh words are dire punishments. Sometimes, although very rarely, physical punishment is used. In all but the most exceptional circumstances it is in the dog's self-interest to allow herself to be trained simply because trained dogs almost invariably enjoy safer and more secure lives.

Food is a powerful reward – so powerful that some dogs will forget they are being trained in order to get it. In these circumstances people should instead use touch as their reward. Different touches mean different things. A simple pat or stroke is all that is needed when a dog is rewarded for good work. Words of praise work well too, but not as well as food or touch. Using positive rewards is a far better way to train a dog than using punishing discipline.

When dogs develop behaviour problems, however, discipline is needed. Nefarious behaviour like sheep-chasing can only be altered by discipline so powerful that it is greater than the thrill the dog gets from the chase. This is one of the rare situations where, with professional help, people might use a shock collar on a dog. For less serious crimes, verbal intimidation, unexpected frights from noises, and physical isolation for two minutes at most are profoundly effective and frequently successful methods to reinforce training.

31. People plan to train me to be aggressive. How will they do it?

In some primitive places pain is still used to train dogs to be aggressive. Through inflicting pain the human makes the dog associate that pain with whatever he is meant to show aggression towards. This is one way that people train dogs to fight each other. Unscrupulous and inhumane people also use this method to train dogs to be aggressive towards strangers.

Enlightened trainers, and this includes most police forces, train dogs to bark aggressively on command and to retrieve rather than to attack. Initially the dog is trained to retrieve an object, frequently an arm-shaped object. He does so with relish and is rewarded by the handler. He then progresses to be trained to retrieve the arm while it is still attached to a human. On command the attack dog leaps at the arm, brings it to the ground where it is easier to handle, then tries to drag it back to his handler. The great advantage of using 'retrieve' to train a dog to be aggressive is that his aggression is always on tap, ready to be turned on or off at the command of his handler. Because it isn't true offensive aggression, the dog remains safe with people as long as he is not commanded to retrieve. Of course police dog handlers have their own egos to satisfy, so they often use the work 'attack' rather than 'retrieve', but that is really a case of semantics.

32. I love chasing sheep but I'm told the farmer has a gun and the right to use it on me. How can I stop behaving like some wild animal?

It is difficult to stop doing what nature intended you to do. The thrills are so enormous, and the rewards so magnificent, that only the most dramatic intervention will stop sheep-chasing.

Dogs instinctively chase anything that moves, and sheep are so defenceless and so dumb that they make perfect victims. Their rapid movements when fearful bring out the primitive in many canines. Dogs who have never before harmed even a grasshopper suddenly feel a deep-seated urge to chase and bite. In a matter of minutes the gentlest of human companions can leave war-like carnage throughout a field, tearing and disembowelling his way through a flock.

Shepherds know that early learning is the best method of prevention, which is why they sometimes put sheepdog pups in a pen with a protective ewe and her lambs. Nothing is as awesome as a mother protecting her young, and a pup quickly learns never to bite, even playfully, and to leave *all* sheep alone. When dogs are near sheep they should always be kept on leads. If a dog has chased sheep in the past, only the most dramatic form of retraining will work. The thrill of the chase must be countermanded by such strong discipline that a dog will think twice about chasing again. This is one of the very few instances where people should consider getting professional assistance to use a remote control shock collar to help eliminate this lethal pursuit.

33. I enjoy tug-of-war but people won't play it with me any more because I get angry if I don't win. What are other good games I can play with them?

Tug-of-war is not a good game to play with a dominant dog who always wants to be the winner, because when she does win she carves a notch on her gun and moves up the pecking order of the pack. This type of game is fine to play with less dominant dogs but only as long as humans always win.

The best games leave humans in control. A simple and effective one is hide-and-seek. This can be played both indoors and out. Either an object or a person is hidden and the dog is then asked to find it. If an object with a strong odour, such as a rubber toy, is hidden, people can rely upon the dog's nose to find it, but they should shout encouragement when she gets near. Hiding people is more difficult but equally effective, as it stimulates the dog's mind to think about where potential hiding places might be. This provides good mental exercise for the dog while at the same time reinforcing her position as a member of the extended pack.

Some dogs play this game professionally. Throughout Europe and North America specially trained squads of hide-and-seekers are on call in the event of avalanche, earthquake or mountain accident. These dogs play the game exactly the same way, following air scent until they find their quarry.

34. Can toys really be intellectually stimulating?

Good toys provide mental and physical stimulation, but the best mimic reality.

Balls, frisbees and eccentrically bouncing 'kongs' are all 'chase' toys. Just as a dog will chase a potential meal, she chases these objects as they try to escape. The most realistic escapers are kongs. Because of their odd shape, they bounce this way and that unexpectedly, just as a rabbit would run. This provides real life exercise for the dog for, rather than running in a straight line, she must be constantly alert to changes of direction.

Toys with squeakers are for killing. The dog often pounces upon these and gives them a quick chew – just as she would do to a mouse.

Hard toys, like nylon rings and rawhide wraps, are for chewing. These exercise the teeth and gums. The front incisor teeth scrape, the large canine teeth hold, and the side molar teeth crush. Few dogs ever get a chance to do these perfectly natural things with food because their meals come out of packages. An additional advantage of this type of toy is that it teaches physical dexterity. Dogs learn to be so nimble with their fore-paws that some people swear they have thumbs.

Finally, there are tug-of-war toys. People enjoy playing with these, not realising that dogs play with them not for intellectual stimulation but simply to win and to show authority over people. All toys remain the property of people. Tug-of-war toys in particular must always be given back to the owners at the end of a game.

35. What early training should my pups have to ensure they grow up to be all-rounders?

From as early an age as possible pups should have all their senses routinely stimulated. They should meet a variety of different animals and people of all sizes. They should travel in cars and walk through pedestrian traffic. Occasionally they should be left alone for a few hours, but they should also be invited to people's parties. The more they experience between birth and twelve weeks of age, the larger their brains will grow and the greater will be the number of interconnections between cells in their brains.

Pups don't have the option of picking who their mothers will be, but mothers do imprint a whole range of behaviours on their pups. Unsure mothers are more likely to produce whining pups, while stern disciplinarians are more likely to produce more introverted progeny. What makes early puppyhood so completely different from early human childhood is that pups are taken away from their mothers and raised by another species. The disadvantage is that it interferes with natural learning; the advantage is that people can teach pups more than their mothers ever could.

Early stimulation of the senses means that a dog is less likely to be frightened by the new or unusual when he is older. That is why dogs raised in cities are almost always less fearful of strangers or strange situations than dogs raised in rural areas. All-rounders should start learning about life – under human supervision – as soon as they want to start exploring.

36. I have heard recently that some people hold puppy parties. What do pups do at them?

A puppy party is really canine kindergarten run by professionals. At kindergarten pups learn how to behave with other pups, how to behave with people, and how to use their senses. Only dogs under a certain age, usually sixteen weeks, are invited to these parties, although each dog is accompanied by her human.

Veterinarians sometimes organise these events and might use more academic words to describe them, such as 'young canine socialisation classes', but the objectives are the same. Pups who have been taken away from their natural litters are brought together weekly with other similarly disadvantaged dogs so that they can continue to learn young dog behaviour from each other. Older dogs are excluded because they are more likely to dominate the parties. At each weekly event pups continue to learn their canine social graces; one of the most important is how to inhibit their bite naturally. They play with other pups who, using perfectly understandable dog language, tell biters when they are biting too hard.

People actively participate in puppy parties too. They bring snack food along with them and give it to other pups when these pups respond to a 'sit' command. This teaches pups that strange people can be quite nice and should also be obeyed. Pups can start partying as soon as they have had their first visit to the veterinarian and are passed as healthy and fit.

37. How much daily exercise should I have? Should I run free or remain on a lead?

The amount of exercise a dog requires varies with his age, breed and early experience. It does not depend on his size: some large or giant dogs need much less exercise than medium, small or even miniature dogs. Once a dog has been fully trained to 'stay' and 'come' on command, he should enjoy having his daily exercise off his lead.

Dogs are inveterate and keen observers of nature. Given the opportunity, a typical dog prefers spending his time outdoors listening to bird song, watching bugs and smelling any scents that waft his way. Just like humans, many dogs act as if they are slightly distanced from the raw naturalness of the world around them, as though they themselves are of a higher and more dignified order. Other dogs are much more urbane in their wants: when offered the choice of lush green grass or a warm sofa on which to while away their lives, they choose the latter.

Homebodies don't need less exercise than green dogs: both need to exercise their bodies fully each day, preferably by running. Ideally dogs should visit different places for their exercise because new vistas are more stimulating. New sights, sounds and smells are invigorating. However, people should be more careful when letting dogs off their leads in these new settings. Fast-growing, big-boned dogs should also see Question 94.

38. What are the best types of collar, harness and lead for me?

A dog's wardrobe varies with her age, breed and general behaviour. Rolled leather collars are excellent because they are unlikely to damage the fur on the neck, although soft, flat nylon collars are almost equally gentle to the fur. Poorly made flat leather collars with rough edges are likely to wear down neck fur; heavy metal collars can do the same. A couple of human fingers should fit under a properly tightened collar. On this garment a dog should wear her necessary identification, including name, telephone number and, where legislation requires it, her vaccination status.

A harness can be better than a collar, especially for thick-necked breeds like pugs or for Yorkshire terriers who sometimes have delicate windpipes. A horse halter-like apparatus is ideal for boisterous or unreliable dogs. The lead is attached to the top of the harness so that there is no pressure on the neck if the dog pulls either forward or back; the lead is attached under the chin on the dog halter, which means that if the dog unexpectedly lunges forward, the momentum pulls her nose down towards the ground and shuts her jaws.

Extendable leads are better than fixed length ones but only if people use them properly. When walking to or from the exercise area, these leads should be locked in a short lead position, but once the dog and her human reach the designated area, the extension can be let out, allowing the dog to explore safely. With good training, the sensible canine can then be released.

39. How can I train people to play fetch with me?

People really like playing fetch with dogs so it isn't difficult to train them. A natural inclination by both parties is necessary, however. Slothful and sedentary people and dogs are not interested in this game. Nor are scent-obsessed dogs, which is why it is more difficult to train a nosey bloodhound than a fawning Labrador.

Retrievable objects should be easy to throw and should fit neatly and safely in a dog's mouth. Tennis balls are ideal for all but the smallest dogs because they are firm yet soft and unlikely to cause damage. Golf balls, although an ideal size for small dogs, are too hard and if caught in flight can break a dog's teeth. Kongs are excellent because they bounce so erratically. Frisbees should only be used with lightweight dogs; heavyset or overweight dogs can tear leg ligaments by jumping high in the air to capture sailing frisbees.

The sensible dog drops an object at a person's feet and kindly but firmly requests that person to throw it. If the dog is a dedicated chewer, she should be on an extended lead and the object should be thrown only a short distance. That way, if the dog does not bring back the object but settles down for a chew instead, she can be reeled in and rewarded with a snack or a stroke for releasing it. It takes most dogs only a very short time to realise that it is more fun to retrieve and return than to retrieve and chew. Verbal rewards then take over, and the training of both parties is complete.

40. When I'm on my leash I want to pull, but when I'm off it I'm content to walk quietly by my person's side. What is it about leashes that makes me behave this way?

For every action there is an equal and opposite reaction. Dogs understand basic physics, so when they feel tension on their lead they simply lean against it. The result is a spluttering dog walking on his hind legs and an exasperated person walking on her heels.

This is an almost inevitable problem if a dog is allowed to lead and is why training him to 'heel' or to walk beside his human is so effective. Instead of holding the lead with one hand, allowing the dog to pull forward, the person should hold it with two hands, one at the top of the lead and the other in the middle, so that the lead is not going up but rather across her body and the dog is beside and slightly behind her. This means that there are no longer any equal and opposite forces. There is nothing for the dog to pull against, and he has no opportunity to pull forward or back.

With no tension on the lead, and using food or toys to get his attention, the person should say the dog's name and start walking. Most dogs will move too. They get rewarded with strokes and words like 'good dog'. If the dog tries to move forward, the person gives a sharp jerk – not a pull – to the lead. Better yet, she steps in front of the dog and confounds him, then starts again. Dogs pull on the lead only because they feel restricted. Most canines enjoy walking with other pack members and will do so obligingly when not restrained.

41. How can I overcome my fear of people?

Fear is partly inherited and partly learned, but it is a firmly set reaction by the time a pup is only a few months old. If a dog is fearful of all people, he needs calm gentling from several people before he can overcome his general worry. If only one person is responsible for retraining him, he will lose his fear with that person but retain it with others.

Unfortunately, a dog who has not been handled by people while he is still a pup will always be frightened by people generally. There is little that can be done. If he has learned fear through human abuse, people should at first avoid both eye and physical contact with him. When he is hungry he should be spoken to soothingly and gently, offered food frequently and become accustomed to the benign presence of humans. And if he sees other dogs enjoying human companionship so much the better; as his fear of people breaks down and he starts to think of them as leaders and providers, his jealousy will develop when he sees other dogs getting enjoyment from physical comfort. He will want his share of attention.

After a short while eye contact can be made. People should remain with the dog while he eats and should continue to utter gentle words. Food is such a powerful reward that the fearful dog might even learn to 'sit' on command for it. The dog will soon willingly come closer and allow himself to be touched. This is the final breakthrough. If several people are involved in reducing his fear, he will realise all the more readily that humans are not as frightening as he once thought.

CHAPTER FOUR

Sex

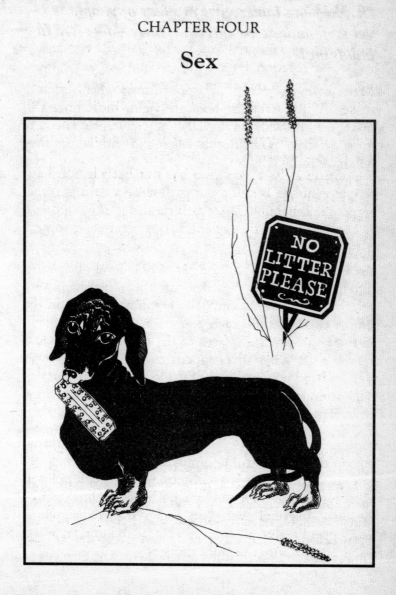

42. Why are males always so interested in sex yet us females only intermittently interested in indulging?

Males of most species are opportunists when it comes to sex. If the circumstances are right, most dogs will mate readily with any available female. Females are more selective. They decide when and with whom they will have sex.

Hormones are responsible for these different attitudes. Day after day males have a relatively constant level of male hormone circulating in their bodies, although the level of hormone might increase a little as daylight gets longer in springtime. A dog's interest in sex remains virtually as constant as his level of circulating male hormone. Females, on the other hand, are relatively inactive, hormonally speaking, except on the one or two occasions each year when the pituitary gland in the brain sends messages to the ovaries to make and release eggs. When this happens, the female experiences a short-lived increase in the female hormone oestrogen. This stimulates her interest in sex and peaks at the time of ovulation.

Curious studies have suggested that human females are more likely to have extramarital affairs around the time they ovulate and their oestrogen levels are highest. It is certainly true that female dogs are most willing to mate immediately after they ovulate, but even then the female will be selective about who her mate will be. Both before and after her oestrogen surge she will decline, sometimes forcefully, any male sexual advances.

43. Why can't I control my promiscuous desire to sleep with people, even strangers?

Some dogs are so lacking in fear of humans that they want to snuggle up to any person they meet. To them all people are generous, magnanimous, warm, caring, door-opening, ball-throwing, can-opener-understanding comforters. They are treat offerers, ticklers and soothers. They offer no harm, and all of them are potential leaders.

Top dogs don't often sleep around. The higher up the ladder a dog thinks he ranks, the less likely he is to crawl into bed with a stranger – or even with his own humans for that matter. Any dog who thinks people are powerful – not just the lowest ranking – is likely to accept a perfect stranger into his pack and fawn over that person.

Members of some breeds such as Alaskan malamutes, chow-chows and huskies think this behaviour is unnecessary, while members of other breeds, such as German shepherds, Labradors and most small breeds, revel in the experience.

As a general rule, females are more likely to sleep around than males. Although it is only a slight tendency, they naturally seek out and enjoy physical contact with other members of their pack, which means they are more likely to roll over to be tickled, paw their owners for attention and creep onto human beds if they can get away with it. This is perfectly natural for the sex that nurtures and enjoys the feeling of contact comfort provided by a litter of pups.

44. People get quite embarrassed. Can you tell me why I am a compulsive flasher and why I prefer revealing myself to people rather than to other dogs?

This form of behaviour is a product of both hormones and learning. Only males flash and usually only when excited. It is a quite normal adolescent activity, but some dogs enjoy doing it so much they continue to expose themselves even in old age.

One of the byproducts of domestication is that a dog becomes sexually mature long before he reaches emotional maturity. Wolves reach both at the same time, at about two years of age, while dogs become adults emotionally at that age but are sexually active well over a year earlier. These youngsters suddenly find that an appendage that served only one purpose now has other uses; they don't know exactly what they are, so they experiment.

Most of these dogs never have the opportunity of seeing – let alone smelling – a female in season, so in the absence of female dogs people can be quite arousing. Humans like touching dogs and playing with them, not realising that touching and playing are essential and arousing parts of normal canine sexual foreplay. Natural mating is always preceded by the female teasing the male to the extent that sometimes she even mounts him. If a young dog finds playing and horsing around with people sexually stimulating, it quite easily becomes a learned and self-perpetuating behaviour. Most dogs flash less once they are emotionally mature.

45. Should I practise safe sex and use contraceptives?

Dogs naturally practise safe sex in that both sexes routinely wash their genitals immediately after each coupling. But there are situations where human help can make sex even safer.

In various parts of the world, but especially in North America, an unpleasant infection called Brucella can be sexually transmitted. Although this disease is apparent when it causes a fever, swollen glands and painful joints, not all dogs that carry the bacteria become clinically ill. Both males and females can be apparently healthy but still act as silent carriers, unwittingly transmitting the infection when they have sex. In the United States this is one of the most common causes of canine infertility. There is no vaccine to prevent Brucellosis, but stud dogs should be blood-tested every three months, and people should make sure that any females that studs mate with have been blood-tested just before mating.

Contraception is another matter entirely. Females can choose between two medical forms of contraception: the needle or the pill. Both of these methods prevent her from ovulating and so are almost foolproof forms of contraception, because if she doesn't ovulate, she won't mate either. For safety reasons the pill or its equivalent of daily contraceptive drops in the food are preferable to long-acting injections. All of these methods might increase the risk of womb infection later in life.

46. How can I become a stud dog?

Stud dogs must be good-looking pure-breds willing to charge a fee for sex. In order to become one, a dog must show that he has extra special aptitudes or abilities. Unfortunately, in most countries all this means is that he is a successful beauty contest winner – that he wins prizes at dog shows.

Ideally a stud dog should have several qualifying characteristics: a good personality, intelligence, excellent conformation and freedom from inherited defects or diseases. This is not always the case. Many kennel clubs don't register known inherited defects, such as a family history of blindness or arthritis, and carriers of these problems have gone on to breed so extensively that they have virtually ruined some breeds.

'Your place or mine' never enters the stud dog's mind. Although he always offers sex on tap, he performs best on his own turf. Sometimes he becomes so accustomed to sex only in his own home that he needs to see and stand on his own special mat before he becomes aroused.

Although it might sound thrilling, some stud dogs lead dull and sedentary lives. Other than when they are at their beauty contests or having sex with complete strangers, they often spend their days incarcerated in their kennels, unable to experience the day-to-day joys of being some person's close companion. It might sound like heaven, but being a stud has drawbacks too.

47. I was minding my own business yesterday, simply having a sniff around in the park, when I was approached by a stranger with whom I consented to have sex. Now I worry that I am pregnant. What can I do?

A pregnancy is very likely in such a situation, so a visit to the vet is necessary. A female dog will only permit mating if she has ovulated recently. This means that dog matings are far more likely to produce offspring than, say, human matings. (Humans may mate like rabbits but most of these matings are for social bonding rather than reproduction. Rabbits and dogs mate for reproduction only.)

Implantation of fertilised eggs can be inhibited if the female is given an injection of female hormone at the right time. If it is given too soon or too late after mating, implantation occurs; once that has happened abortion is much more difficult. There are chemical abortion methods but these are quite unsatisfactory. At this stage only a hysterectomy will terminate the pregnancy.

One of the drawbacks of the morning-after injection is that it puts the female's cycle back to day one. This means that another ovulation will usually take place ten to fourteen days later, so she must be extra vigilant that she does not fall under the spell of a handsome stranger again.

48. If I do become pregnant, how will I know? Should I change any of my habits? How long will my pregnancy last?

Some dogs don't realise they are pregnant and behave quite normally until they go into labour, but most seem to realise a few weeks after mating. This is when a dog should start reducing her physical activity a little.

A typical pregnancy lasts around sixty-three days, but it is not until thirty-five days after mating that her nipples become prominent and her abdomen visibly enlarges – the first overt signs that she is carrying a litter. If people gently feel her abdomen about twenty-eight days after conception, they should be able to count the golf ball-like fetuses in her womb. This is difficult to do on tense or fat dogs, and in these circumstances ultrasound is a sophisticated alternative. This method of pregnancy diagnosis is most accurate when it is used twenty to twenty-five days after mating. Each little golf ball-like fetus shows up clearly on the video screen. Ultrasound diagnosis continues to be easy later on in the pregnancy, but because the developing pups grow so quickly it's more difficult to count them. By forty-two days there is calcium in the developing pups' bones, so the litter shows up quite dramatically on X-ray.

At about forty-nine days, the dog's mammary glands start to engorge, filling with milk, and at fifty-six days she might start producing a watery discharge from her nipples. This means that milk will soon be in production. During these latter stages of pregnancy, the expectant canine should remember that she isn't as agile as she used to be. Her centre of gravity has changed and her unborn litter acts like a pendulum, reducing her ability to take tight corners at high speed, something she will still want to do if sufficiently stimulated.

Because a hormonal 'phantom' pregnancy is the normal conclusion to each and every reproductive cycle, urine tests are useless at diagnosing a pregnancy. The hormone of pregnancy is there even when the dog is not pregnant. Some sophisticated blood tests have been developed, but even these are not very accurate. Fortunately most females simply know when they are carrying pups, and reduce their activity and the possible risk to their unborn babies.

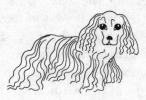

49. I am soft and sensual. Are there any benefits in my having a litter or is it better for me to be spayed?

Unlike humans, even the softest, most sensual dog does not have a life-long need to nurture. The benefits of motherhood to dogs are different from those to people.

Strong social bonds develop between a mother and her pups, bonds that help her young to survive. She feeds them, comforts them and will fight to the death to protect them – to a point. That point is reached when they are still very young. It starts when their pinpoint-sharp teeth bite when they suckle. It hurts and she either disciplines the biter or walks away. That, in fact, is the reason why the pups' teeth are so sharp in the first place, for this is the first stage in a natural separation process that breaks down maternal bonds.

Over the next few weeks, as the pups grow and as the mother's milk-producing hormone level drops, the role of the pup changes from dependant to competitor. The litter becomes a pack and, although the mother retains authority, the day will come when a grown pup challenges her for rank. By this time virtually all maternal feelings will have disappeared and have been replaced by competitive ones.

Spaying can interfere with a dog's gentleness but only when a female already has a tendency to be dominantly aggressive. Soft and gentle dogs remain that way after spaying, but dominant females might become more so if they are spayed and no longer experience the 'softening' effect of twice yearly surges of female hormone.

50. Will neutering make me fat and boring?

If calories are not watched, neutering can definitely make a dog fat, but not boring.

In both males and females the sex cycle uses up calories. Dogs obviously burn up energy when looking for sex, but they also use calories to make eggs and sperm. Both the oestrous cycle in females and sex-related aggression and territory patrol in males are energy-consuming. When a dog is neutered these energy demands drop. The amount of food eaten should drop too.

Neutering does alter certain male behaviours, but the changes are interesting rather than boring. Most neutered males don't feel as great a need to urine-mark their territories. Less urine-marking makes them more appealing human companions, so they find they are disciplined less and played with more. Similarly, neutering reduces vagrancy and sex-related male-to-male aggression. Less of these behaviours means less danger. Neutering does not diminish any other form of aggression or reduce a dog's natural inquisitiveness, it simply pushes sex down from the top priority a dog has and allows other activities like hunting, tracking, retrieving, or playing games to become more prominent.

If a dog is to be neutered, people should make sure that they watch that dog's calories for several months after the operation. A simple rule is to reduce calorie intake by ten per cent immediately after neutering. A drop of twenty-five per cent is quite normal but only becomes necessary if weight is gained.

51. Why do I try to have sex with everything I see: cushions, knees, cats, anything? Am I simply oversexed?

This is the behaviour of the young, the oversexed and the inexperienced. Very often, just as with flashing, these activities are those of the human's companion who never has an opportunity to direct his sexual advances at the real thing.

Most dogs reach puberty in the privacy of a human household. Although there are many multiple dog families, the majority of dogs live without in-house canine companionship. This means that when their sexual apparatus first needs testing there are no other dogs to test it on, so they choose the next best thing, a person, a cushion or even a cat.

Masturbating is a perfectly normal canine activity but some people find it both offensive and disturbing, especially if a dog chooses to perform either on or in the presence of a human visitor. Some dogs have their favourite cushion and will carry it off to a quiet corner for a little stimulation, while others, depending upon their size, prefer human elbows or knees. Stuffed toys appear to be divinely designed sex aids to certain dogs.

A stern 'NO!' from a person, combined with a minute's isolation in a quiet and empty room each time a dog masturbates, will so reduce the dog's enjoyment that the behaviour can be completely eliminated within a few weeks. If a young dog is not reprimanded when he first starts masturbating, it soon becomes a firmly ingrained habit and is more difficult to overcome.

52. Why do I lust after castrated males but show no interest in females even when they flaunt themselves at me?

Homosexuality is common among a wide variety of mammals, but lusting after castrates might not mean a desire for sex. If a dog were genuinely homosexual, he would prefer trying to mate with males rather than with females. This is very uncommon. Some males are completely indifferent to females, and take no notice of them even when the ladies lasciviously body-bash and flaunt their posteriors. Uninterested dogs are often very human-orientated and lack any experience in mating, but they are uninterested in males too.

Some dogs try to mount castrated males for two interrelated reasons. The first is that they have tried to mount everything else before, unsuccessfully. They've tried to mount females but have been driven away; they've tried to mount males and have been bitten; but when they tried to mount a castrate they were not driven off and so carried on. This becomes a lesson learned.

The connected second reason is dominance. Mounting and pelvic thrusting is obviously sexual but it is also symbolically dominant. A dog will mount and pelvic thrust upon another dog regardless of sex simply to show who is boss. Even females will sometimes behave this way. Mounting a castrated male might be a completely sexual act in some circumstances, but in others it is merely a show of authority.

53. Recently after I had sex I got stuck. It took half an hour before we could separate. I felt like a jerk. What happened?

Getting stuck is simply a natural part of mating, and is called 'tying'. It ensures that the ejaculated semen remains in the vagina, and at the same time it prevents any other dog from mating with the receptive female.

The male has a special apparatus on his penis that swells balloon-like after he has mated successfully. At the same time, muscles just inside the female's vulva clamp down so that there is virtually a watertight seal, like a silicone plug in a glass bottle. The male's swelling, the bulbourethral gland, sometimes enlarges when a dog becomes sexually excited, and he can't withdraw his penis back into the sheath. As long as it doesn't become too dry, he will be able to withdraw it ten to fifty minutes later, about the length of time that a natural tie with a female lasts.

During the time that the couple are stuck together, the male often lifts his hind leg over her back so that they stand tail to tail, looking faintly ridiculous and even glum as they stare at the ground or dream canine dreams. It might look dumb, but this is a sensible precaution, because tail-to-tail both dogs can see and meet with danger coming from any direction while their natural defences are lowered by their compromising situation.

54. Why is it that after each of my seasons I become irritable and snappy with other dogs and people and sometimes produce milk even though I'm not pregnant?

All of these behaviours are caused by hormonal changes that occur after each season. Unlike most other mammals, a dog will always undergo the hormone changes of pregnancy after every single oestrous cycle regardless of whether she is pregnant or not.

After eggs are released into the fallopian tubes, the empty craters on the ovaries start producing progesterone, the hormone of pregnancy. This is an efficient way to ensure that the womb is ready to receive fertilised eggs, but rather than turning off production when fertilised eggs are not present, the ovaries continue to produce progesterone for the full two-month period that a real pregnancy would last. This hormone affects the dog's shape and behaviour. Her taste buds might change, as well as her appetite. She might become more sedentary, preferring to relax and doze rather than to play hard. She will often seek out secluded den-like resting places under tables and behind sofas. She might become possessive over toys or other objects and carry them around as if they were pups.

In the latter stages of her false pregnancy a female might produce milk, sometimes so much that she needs medication to reduce its production. And she can develop maternal aggression, one of the most fearsome forms of canine authority, and will possessively protect her den and her 'pups'. Fortunately the entire cycle is self-limiting and ends two months after it begins.

55. People want me to mate with my father. Won't that produce a litter of deformed idiots?

Incest can be dangerous for the unborn, although it is the way that many breeds were originally developed. People use inbreeding and line breeding today mostly to perpetuate physical characteristics in their dogs. If, in a litter, there is one male pup with cobalt blue eyes, that pup might be mated back with his mother to try to perpetuate this new eye colour. If, in the litter, one male and one female have this unique feature, the brother and sister might be mated together when they reach sexual maturity.

These forms of breeding accentuate obvious physical characteristics but they are just as likely to concentrate 'bad' genes. Bad genes are always lurking about but are infrequent enough so that they seldom meet up with the other bad gene to make the pair that are necessary to create a problem. Haemophilia, the blood-clotting disorder, is rare in dogs because the gene that carries it is 'recessive' or infrequent. Haemophilia virtually never occurs in mixed breed dogs. But by breeding selectively for certain traits, and in creating specific breeds, humans have accentuated in these breeds the deleterious genes that cause haemophilia. Just as with the former Russian royal family, inbreeding has made breeds like the St Bernard more prone to bleeding disorders. Rather than idiocy, bleeding disorders are more representative of the true problems of inbreeding.

56. Why did I eat my newborn babies? Have I been watching too many horror movies?

Cannibalism is rare but not unknown in dogs. It occurs most frequently in breeds once bred for fighting. It is more likely to be a behaviour of the inexperienced or nervous mother than of the experienced or relaxed female.

The risk of cannibalism is greater after a Caesarean section than after natural birth, so people should always carry out a twenty-four-hour watch on pups delivered in this way. If a female wakes up from an anaesthetic in a place with strange odours, surrounded by a mass of squirming small animals she has never seen before, she can behave in an unexpected manner.

Even with a routine delivery, some mothers get carried away, exaggerating natural birthing behaviours into excessive ones. Instead of chewing off the umbilical cord and eating the afterbirth, they eat the afterbirth, then the umbilical cord and then the pup.

Cannibalism is an unpleasant but biologically normal method of birth control in mammals such as hamsters and mice. It is not normal yet should still be anticipated in some dogs. People should carry out round-the-clock watches for several days on Staffordshire and English bull terriers, American Staffs and pugs. Only when a mother has relaxed into a placid grooming and feeding routine, and after the umbilical cord has shrivelled, is it safe to give up the constant watch.

57. *People want me to mate to teach their children about sex. Is this fair?*

No, it isn't. If people want to offer sex lessons for their children, they can certainly provide the information in a more relevant way than having their kids watch two dogs mate.

Virtually everywhere in the world there is a surplus of unwanted pups. Any canine pregnancy should be planned not as a lesson for children but because people would like to have pups from that specific mating. Good homes should be available to the resulting progeny.

That doesn't mean that the cycle of life is not instructive for children; it certainly is. Children can learn about reproduction by understanding how conception occurs and what happens at birth. It is a pretty poor lesson in sexuality or caring, however. If dogs are models, children soon learn that sex is simply slam bam without even a 'Thank you ma'am', and that males have no part to play in child rearing.

Because dogs are kept in a controlled human environment, people are responsible for ensuring that their reproduction is controlled too. This means that the welfare of the products of any mating should be the primary concern.

CHAPTER FIVE

Diet

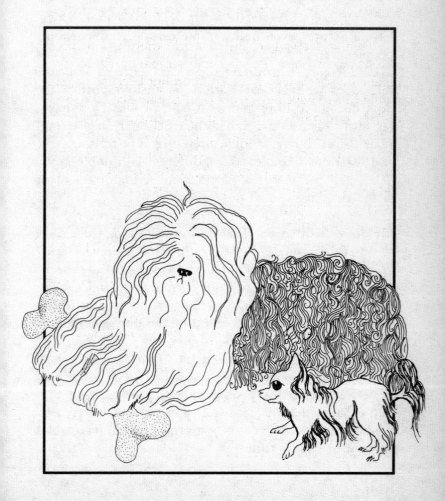

58. I crave rabbit droppings. Horse manure makes my mouth water. I can't resist dipping into the cat's litter tray. I even eat my own droppings. Am I sick?

All of these are perfectly normal canine habits. Dogs have a natural, even healthy, interest in droppings, but people often find this interest quite disgusting.

Unlike cats, who prefer their food as fresh as possible, dogs willingly eat carrion. Taste is important to dogs but not as important as it is to people. Dogs have far fewer taste buds; rather than delicately registering sweet, sour, bitter or salty, they probably register general reactions like pleasant, indifferent and unpleasant. The smell and texture of food is more important than taste – droppings smell and feel divine.

Manure, especially herbivore manure, is nutritious for dogs. It often contains nutrients and enzymes that are useful in canine digestion. Puppies, especially fast-growing puppies, usually first eat droppings as an experiment. They get pleasure from finding them and tasting them. If the exercise is rewarding, and that can mean either the droppings taste good or the pup gets lots of attention from people when he behaves this way, the initial experiment becomes a habit. Sometimes dogs will eat droppings because they have a lack of digestive enzymes. If this is the case, people should augment the dog's diet with either enzyme supplements or enzyme-containing foods such as pineapple, pumpkin, vegetable marrow or papaya fruit.

59. Sometimes I pass such foul wind that even I leave the room. How can I control it?

Intestinal gas is produced by gas-forming bacteria, and the number of bacteria will vary with the food that is eaten. Altering the diet is the most sensible way for a dog to become more socially acceptable.

Flatulence is often associated with eating legumes like beans and peas, but a wide variety of different foods will stimulate these bacteria to multiply in a dog's gastrointestinal system. In fact, there are no hard and fast rules about which diets make dogs windy. In theory, diets high in roughage should do so, while high protein diets should not. In practice, however, high protein, all meat diets can turn some dogs into gas factories, while poor quality, high roughage diets don't.

Antibiotics sometimes cause dogs to pass foul wind because they upset the bacterial balance in the gut. When this happens, feeding yoghurt that contains 'nice' live bacteria can rectify the problem. In other circumstances dogs should alter their eating habits, trying various combinations of foods, each for a couple of weeks at a time, to find out which ones result in the best formed stools with the least gas. If a dog wants to stick to the diet he likes, live yoghurt or special 'nice' bacteria-containing nutritional aids can be mixed in his food as supplements to aid digestion and improve social acceptability.

60. Why do I hate sharing and always want what other dogs have rather than what I am given?

Jealousy is a natural part of dog behaviour, and jealousy over food is one of its most common manifestations. Even when one dog has the most magnificent, succulent, meaty, marrowy bone that ever existed, if he sees another dog with a shrivelled insignificant drumstick he will still feel the urge to have that too. This attitude is an integral part of his pack behaviour. In the pack, if you share you end up getting less, but if you take you get more, become physically stronger and advance towards leadership in the pecking order.

Pet dogs show their authority in the same way: takers are more dominant than sharers. Pet dogs have another excuse for their dominant behaviour. People are included in their natural inclination to want what other dogs have – to most pet dogs, people *are* other dogs – and the food people have smells and tastes an awful lot better than what they have in their own bowls. So when a family settles down for their meal, the dog has two valid reasons for preferring what the rest of the family is eating to what has been given to him.

The simple and effective method people should use to overcome this problem is never to feed a dog from the table and always to feed him after they have eaten. If he sees people eat first, he intuitively knows that they are unassailable pack leaders, and leaders always eat first. This will reduce his dominance and natural inclination to have what people have. It won't reduce his desire to have what another dog has, however, so when two dogs are given bones, to reduce the possibility of conflict, they should eat them in separate rooms.

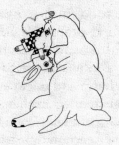

61. People feed me the same things at the same time day after day. Shouldn't I have a more varied diet?

If a diet is perfectly well balanced there is no harm in a dog eating the same food for her entire life. This puts a lot of faith in the food preparer's ability to make sure every vitamin, trace mineral, essential fatty acid and amino acid is present in just the right quantity, so varying the diet does no harm and might even do good.

Dogs often get very settled in their ways. They enjoy routine and this can include knowing that they get fed with a certain food at a certain time each day. Frequency is quite important. Anatomically dogs are built to gorge once or twice a week and then live off the large reserve sitting in the stomach. Given their preference, they enjoy eating more frequently, at least once or twice a day. This frequency is set up early in life. Later on it will be easy to increase, but disquieting for the dogs if it is reduced. From a nutritional viewpoint the number of meals each day is irrelevant: the number of daily calories is the most important factor.

Occasionally changing brands or even the texture of food from dry, soft-moist or canned can be exciting for some dogs but cause diarrhoea in others. An alternative is to stick to what a dog likes but to add a vitamin and mineral supplement to her diet. Nutritionally these are probably quite unnecessary but they taste good, can be used as rewards during training, may fill an unknown gap in her nutritional intake and, when given in recommended amounts, can do no harm.

62. Even though I am well fed, and if anything even a little bit overweight, why do I have this constant need to scavenge?

Scavenging is fun. It is real dog work. It is exciting and rewarding. A dog can use his senses to do what they were meant to do: search, investigate and consume. Like wealthy business people who do deals not because they need more money but because of the thrill of doing deals, dogs scavenge not because they need more food but because of the high that comes from scavenging. That is why even well-fed dogs willingly scavenge.

Boredom is an integral component of scavenging. Working dogs, such as search and rescue, police and guide dogs, who must concentrate their minds on other activities are less likely to scavenge than sedentary couch lizards. For the majority of pet dogs, however, a daily outing to a park or recreation area is the highlight of the day; it is the only time that all the senses can be used to investigate who has been visiting that territory and what food might lie within it.

In the absence of rigorous exercise, food and feeding sometimes become prime objectives in life. Rather than living for exercise, some dogs live for food, and finding it becomes their main reason for being. When this happens, scavenging becomes even more than just self-rewarding, it becomes the reason for living.

63. Why do I have this compulsion to bury bones?

Burying bones is a vestige of the dog's prehistoric past, when she saved food for days of famine. All dogs have the potential to bury bones : ut few realise their ambition.

Many canines only ever see bones on people's dinner plates. They are never given them because of the possible, though often exaggerated, dangers they present. Swallowed bone can produce constipation or even a complete intestinal blockage that can be relieved only through surgery. Boneless dogs still have the same bone-burying urges as other dogs, so they usually bury dog treats, chews and biscuits instead. When a garden isn't available, these deprived dogs try to bury objects in carpets, especially in corners, and frustratingly try to cover the 'buried' object by pushing the carpet with their nose.

Dogs with gardens will bury objects symbolically rather than practically, for they often forget about their buried objects and never dig them up. Some dogs will bury cats or squirrels they have killed, to let them ripen. Wild canines such as foxes bury bird eggs and later dig them up and eat them. Burying food protects it from other scavengers and provides a larder for times of want. Because dogs have lived on human handouts for so long, burying bones has become a symbolic rather than a practical activity.

64. Sometimes I have an urge to graze on grass just like a cow. I thought I was a carnivore. Does this craving mean that I'm really a closet vegetarian?

Although dogs are carnivorous and enjoy meat, they are not, like cats, dependent upon meat for survival. Grazing is perfectly normal, even beneficial.

Grass adds fibre to the diet. This bulks up the intestinal contents and helps it pass through to the far end. Just as with humans, fibre in a dog's diet might be medically beneficial too, reducing the risk of bowel cancer. Rather than graze randomly, many dogs look for very specific grasses or weeds to eat. These herbivorous dogs prefer succulent new dew-covered spring grass to drier older forms. It is like a fresh green salad and the morning dew a bland vinaigrette. Later in the year it is not uncommon for dogs to graze on summer and early autumn berries, especially blackberries. This isn't random behaviour but rather a selective choice on the part of the grazer.

Because they can manufacture essential fatty acids and amino acids themselves, unlike cats, dogs can survive on strictly vegetarian diets, although this is not how they have been designed to live. Vegetable-derived fats and proteins can form the building blocks that are necessary for life, but it is more difficult to ensure a proper balance of nutrients solely from plant rather than from both plant and animal sources. Dogs are really omnivores. They willingly try almost anything and many enjoy a light vegetarian meal on occasion.

65. I have good days and I have bad days. Is my diet related to my swings in mood and behaviour?

There is no concrete evidence that diet is related to dog mood but there is lots of conflicting circumstantial evidence that behaviour is related to what a dog eats. Some people think that certain amino acids, the building blocks of protein, are related to aggression, and by reducing the consumption of these amino acids it is possible to reduce a dog's need to be aggressive. Meat contains these theoretically mind-bending amino acids, so the argument goes that if you reduce the amount of meat a dog eats he will be less aggressive.

Other scientists argue the exact opposite. They say that certain brain chemicals are made from meat-derived amino acids and these chemicals *control* aggression. If these amino acids are absent, then control of predatory aggression is also absent and the dog goes out looking for a meal. Once it has eaten some animal protein that replenishes these amino acids, it turns off his need to kill again.

Whichever theory is true, there is no doubt that poor diet and lethargy are related. If a diet consists of poor quality foods, the intestines, liver and kidneys have to work overtime to cope with the toxic excess of waste products. Energy is sapped and a dog becomes dull, even seemingly depressed. Balanced nutrition helps keep most dogs in prime mental condition.

66. Sometimes I gulp down my food so fast that I forget I've eaten. Is this dangerous?

Humans think it uncouth behaviour to gobble, but in the context of pack mentality it is a perfectly normal, acceptable and beneficial way to eat; for that matter, so is immediately regurgitating a meal then eating it again.

Part of the behavioural baggage that dogs brought with them when they moved from the forest to the fireplace was competitive feeding. 'What you have I want' is one manifestation, while vacuuming food without chewing or seemingly tasting it is another. Throwing large chunks into his mouth, a dog empties his food bowl within seconds, then looks up plaintively at people to ask what magic made it disappear. People think this is absurd behaviour for a lone dog that has never had to compete with other dogs for his food. They forget that as far as the dog is concerned people are simply other large hairless dogs. He feels the need to compete with them even if they never get down on the floor and challenge for the food bowl.

Eating quickly is sometimes followed by regurgitation, but this, too, is normal dog behaviour, especially among females who naturally regurgitate to feed their growing pups. Some dogs eat grass, not as a salad but to help regurgitate food. They do this when they feel stomach discomfort or simply to unload an overworked system.

67. I am a picky eater and will sometimes go for days without food. Is this called anorexia and is it dangerous?

Yes, this is a form of anorexia and, no, it is not dangerous. Dogs are built with large holding tank stomachs and relatively short intestines. Through natural selection large breeds of dogs have evolved to have a generalist's taste in food. They will try anything and eat plenty of it, keeping their holding tanks as full as possible; this is a good ploy for a dog who as a pup has to grow quickly and then as an adult must consume large numbers of calories to maintain his weight. In the survival of the fittest, the least food faddy dogs are the most likely winners.

This form of natural selection pressure has never applied to small breeds of canines. Small breeds evolved from human intervention in dog breeding, with humans helping runts and genetic freaks to survive. Instead of dying early in life or surviving but failing in competition with larger dogs for mating privileges, these small dogs evolved without the natural evolutionary pressure to eat everything available. The result is that food faddiness or anorexia is almost unheard of in large breeds like German shepherds and Labradors but quite common in small breeds like Yorkshire terriers and Chihuahuas.

Anorexia is less likely to occur in dogs from large litters. As pups they learned that if you don't compete you go hungry. This is why some people get down on their hands and knees and pretend they are eating dog food in an attempt to convince a dog to eat.

Anorexia is not as dangerous in dogs as it is in humans because beneath the small dog's demands for special foods lies a wolf's gastrointestinal system and a wolf's common sense that food is necessary for survival. Metabolically speaking, dogs are very well equipped to go without food for considerably longer than people can before their kidneys or other organs become damaged. Historically, the Inuit in northern Canada and Alaska fed their working sled dogs copious amounts of food every four days. These dogs retained robust good health because the feeding pattern was similar to that of the local wolves. Arctic wolf packs successfully kill and gorge on caribou or deer about every four days. Because of their gastrointestinal anatomy, all dogs find it far easier to go without food for several days than people do, but once they are really hungry they will eat what is available.

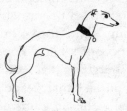

68. Why do people get up and leave the room when I yawn?

Bad breath. Dogs don't mind having bad breath but people find it quite offensive. Although it can be created by the food that is eaten, in most instances bad breath means either mouth or digestion problems, most of which can be overcome.

Dogs smell of the food they eat. If they eat manure or fish, they smell of it. But if there are digestion problems smells can come from the stomach too. These dogs usually burp; if the burped smell is unpleasant it means that bacterial fermentation or other smell-making activities are occurring in the stomach. If this is happening, the diet should be changed.

The most common cause of bad breath is gum inflammation resulting from calculus build-up on teeth. A dog's teeth yellow with age but chewing on skin and bones or brushing his teeth prevents mineral deposits from sticking to them. If a dog doesn't routinely massage his teeth and gums, a scummy slime forms on the gnashers and this thickens and becomes hard. Food catches between the build-up and the gums, bacteria multiply, and the dog's breath turns into a lethal weapon.

Bad breath usually means gum infection, which, in turn, means that each time the halitosis sufferer chews food he pumps bacteria into his bloodstream. While he is healthy and fit his defence system eliminates these germs, but when he is not, these circulating bacteria can produce a generalised infection and are thought to be involved in the most common form of heart disease.

CHAPTER SIX

Travel

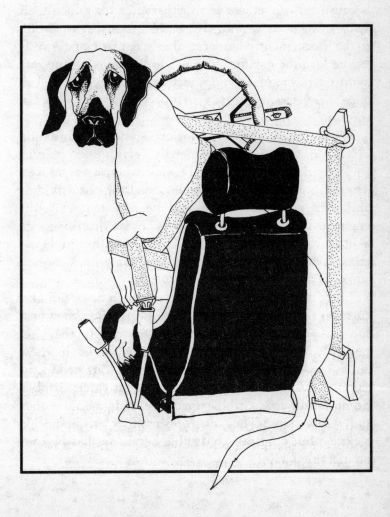

69. Why do I dribble whenever I get in a car?

Dribble is a sign of nausea. If dogs dribble in cars it means they want to be sick.

Motion sickness is common in young pups simply because car movement is an experience for which their sense of balance was not created. All four feet are meant to be permanently under a dog's control and firmly planted on the ground. Just as with humans, if pups are exposed to frequent and short car journeys, their balance mechanism evolves to cope with this type of motion.

Without early learning, motion sickness is more difficult to control. Adult dogs need several weeks' training to learn not to dribble or be sick when a car moves. They should get in a car, be rewarded for not dribbling and then get out. This should be repeated while the engine is running. Rewards follow for no dribbling with a little car movement and eventually with simple car trips. Training can be tedious and sometimes motion sickness tablets are a simple answer.

There are other circumstances in which dogs, tap-like, turn on their saliva glands. Some do it when they hear humans using can openers; others when they see peanuts, vitamin tablets or favourite foods. In these situations dogs expect to be fed so they start producing saliva. This can also be a reason why car riders dribble. Some adult dogs dribble in cars simply because they did so as pups. They no longer suffer from motion sickness but continue to dribble because it has become an ingrained habit.

70. People wear seatbelts when they get in the car. Shouldn't I wear one too?

Dogs are just as likely to be injured in car accidents as people are. Their problem is that most don't know how to release their seatbelts if they have to get out of a car quickly.

A dog should never travel on the front passenger seat of a car unless there are extraordinary reasons for doing so. Without the steering wheel for protection, this is the death seat. In an accident the dog is likely to be thrown forward and suffer substantial injuries.

She is far safer on a back seat. If the car suddenly stops, the dog is thrown against the back of the front seats. Injuries such as fractures are still common, however, because the dog falls into the foot well. Dog seatbelts are harness-like and prevent this type of dangerous forward movement. They attach to standard seatbelt latches and reduce injuries caused when the dog continues to move after the car has stopped.

Nosey and curious back seat drivers, especially small terriers, enjoy climbing under the rear window for the best view. These small dogs become flying missiles when cars stop abruptly. Other canines have convinced people to buy station wagons especially for them. They like being able to get up and go for a little walk while travelling in the car. Firmly secured dog guards between the dog and passenger sections of the vehicle reduce the risk of injury to both parties.

71. I know we are only going to the park, so why do I yap my lungs out, pace back and forth, and do backwards somersaults until we get there?

For some dogs car rides are among the most thrilling events in their lives, not because the ride itself is much fun but because they have learned to associate the trip with the excitement to follow. Often these are house-bound dogs, incarcerated for life in luxurious but boring surroundings. They literally leap for joy when they know they are about to be released from enforced physical and mental solitude for a few minutes.

Overwrought behaviour is boring to people. Constant yapping, pacing and barking is distracting to them and therefore dangerous. Dogs can be trained to be quiet in cars, although this training must be inventive and is sometimes difficult. If there is an empty road nearby and a dog is not wearing a seatbelt, a car driver can shout 'NO BARKING!' and at the same time throw on the car brakes. This has a salutary and arresting effect on many dogs.

Better still, a second person can be employed to silence the canine jabberer. While the driver concentrates on driving, this person gets in with the dog and commands him to sit and be quiet. Because of the chemical changes that occur in the body, hysteria is intensely rewarding in its own way. This is why it can be so difficult to overcome. Theatrics are necessary and can work wonders. If the dog continues to bounce with excitement, an unexpected squirt from a water pistol will get some dogs' attention. Noise-makers work well with others. Yapping must only be disciplined. It should not be rewarded with soothing words, strokes or food, as these only reinforce the activity.

People should not wind up dogs emotionally by telling them in expectant tones where they will be going. Departures should be as calm as possible. During training, if a dog starts barking as soon as he hops in the car, he should be reprimanded and told to get out and go back inside his house. Car entrances are then repeated until he gets in and does not yap. The same exercise is repeated if he barks on the way to the park. The driver turns around and drives back home. If rewards are denied, a dog will learn within weeks to control his vocal urges.

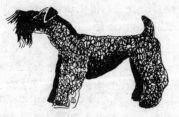

72. I overheard people saying I'm going to be sent to kennels for a week. Friends have told me they are like prisons. What should I expect?

Kennel life is heaven for some dogs and hell for others. Dog-orientated dogs actively enjoy being sentenced to a week or more in kennels. They enjoy seeing, hearing and scenting other dogs. They become more alert, especially if they are permitted to exercise with fellow inmates or even to room with them. Human-orientated dogs, on the other hand, can find forced living with other dogs extremely distasteful. For them, staying in kennels is a bit like an unathletic urban human being forced to go on a survival course.

Good kennels cater for both types of canine personality. Kennel units themselves should have warm indoor facilities as well as connected outdoor runs. They should be designed so that reclusive dogs can retire to secluded areas where they can't be seen, while extravert dogs move to other parts of the kennels where they can see and communicate with other extraverts. This is easily achieved by having a platform in each kennel. Introverts have their beds under the platform, while extraverts spend most of their time on top of it.

Good kennel menus contain a choice of foods, including home-made, individually packaged TV dinners for truly picky eaters. Perhaps most important of all are the staff at the kennels. These people should be thoroughly inspected. The more questions *they* ask about a dog, the more likely they are to be considerate of an individual dog's specific needs and requirements.

73. Wouldn't it be better if people got in a housesitter or I stayed with the neighbours rather than their sending me to a canine Colditz?

These are good sensible alternatives to kennelling. Friends or relatives are sometimes willing to move into people's homes to look after lonesome canines. There are even professional dog sitters who come fully referenced and insured to care for empty homes and their livestock.

Staying with neighbours is a little trickier. Caring for an unfamiliar dog can be difficult and exasperating. A male dog might want to urine-mark his new territory. The temporary carers might not be familiar with the dog's normal sanitary routines, and this could result in unwelcome and unexpected puddles and mess. Only the kindest of neighbours is willing to put up with these inconveniences. The possibility of straying is also dramatically greater when a dog is away from home and not surrounded by a dog-proof perimeter fence. He might even intentionally stray to try to find his way back to his own home.

Looking after an unfamiliar dog is sometimes a greater responsibility than looking after someone's child. If people must choose between leaving a dog with lukewarm neighbours or in a professional kennel, they should choose the latter. As long as the kennel is well designed and operated by people who genuinely enjoy dogs, it is the safer option.

74. I'm an inquisitive dog and would like to explore the world outside my garden. Is there any guaranteed way of my finding my own way home if I stray?

Most dogs that stray get lost and never find their way home. Canines navigate by using all of their senses. They remember sights, sounds and noises. If they don't come across any familiar ones, they get as lost as people do. Some panic and race back and forth not knowing what to do; others apply common sense and embark on a methodical search for anything familiar.

The most methodical dogs will work in ever increasing circles, sniffing ground and air scents for anything they recognise. When a familiar odour is found, they follow it until they recognise where they are.

In almost every country there are stories of dogs finding their way home from hundreds of miles away. These dogs traverse rivers, mountains, deserts, cities, industrial landscapes and superhighways to turn up finally, footsore but happy, on their own doorstep. Occasionally dogs manage to do this and it could be that they have an electromagnetic navigational ability like birds, but it is a one in a million chance. People relish these stories. They want to think that dogs can find their way home because they have enshrined the idea of canine loyalty in human folklore. The sad reality is that dogs get lost more easily than people do and in the absence of identification and human help are unlikely ever to find their way home.

75. What if I lose my dog tag? Are there any sure ways by which I can identify myself?

Dog tags bearing the dog's name and telephone number on permanently worn dog collars are the best means of identification. It is a good idea to have the veterinarian's telephone number on the tag, so that if a lost dog is found and her people are not home, the finders know who to contact for advice or medical attention. All veterinarians provide twenty-four-hour emergency cover, so someone is always available.

Collars and tags go missing so it is a good idea for the dog to carry additional ID on her body. The most common means are tattoos or microchip implants injected under the skin.

Tattooing an identification number in the ear is an easy, painless and cheap method of permanent identification. It works best when it is either part of a national dog registration scheme or is administered by a national organisation such as a kennel club. When a tattoo-numbered dog turns up at a police station or dog shelter, a call to the registration centre identifies the dog and his most recent home address and telephone number.

The high-tech equivalent to tattooing is implanting a tiny transponder under the dog's neck skin. This is done by a simple injection. When a scanner is fanned over the dog, it 'reads' the transponder's information. This form of ID is only useful when all dog shelters and police stations scan dogs for implants. The unexpected bonus is that it is a tamper-proof form of identity in case of disputes.

76. Let's say I get lost, have no identification and end up in a dog shelter. What are my chances of coming out of there alive?

Miserable. Throughout Europe, North America and Australasia, dog shelters are forced to kill millions of dogs every year. Some are killed because they are elderly and unwell, others because they are dangerous, but the vast majority are healthy dogs destroyed simply because they have no ID and no people can be found who want to live with them.

Some charities have a 'no kill' policy. If a dog ends up in one of these dog shelters, he is kept as long as it takes to find a home for him. If he carries no ID but is young, active and intelligent, he might even join a training programme at another charity to become a 'hearing dog' and spend a stimulating life acting as ears for a profoundly deaf person. Otherwise he lingers in kennels built specifically for long-stay inmates, always on show for people who might, one day, want to take him into their own home.

This is the exception rather than the rule. Unidentified dogs usually live for only days, or at the most weeks, after they enter a dog shelter. The luckiest are usually young pure-breds. For some curious reason these are the dogs most likely to be taken into a new home by the generous people who visit dog shelters. It's curious, because pure-breds are certainly no healthier than cross-bred or mongrel dogs. Because selective breeding increases the risk of inherited diseases, pure-breds often suffer from a wider range of possible problems than their less highly bred cousins. Pure-breds are not more intelligent either, although the personality traits of a pure-bred are easier to anticipate because these too can be inherited.

Upon arrival at the shelter dogs get a medical examination and treatment for any existing problems and then go on show. People come and look at them. The wisest dogs put on extra mascara, wag their tails as fast as they can and smile broadly as people pass by, but it is only the luck of the draw that decides which ones find new homes. Because there is such an overwhelmingly large and unending number of unidentified stray dogs, if shelter inmates can't convince people to take them home, they are soon killed to make way for the constant procession of others.

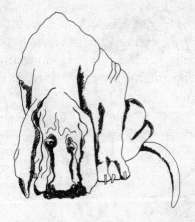

CHAPTER SEVEN

Illness and Disease

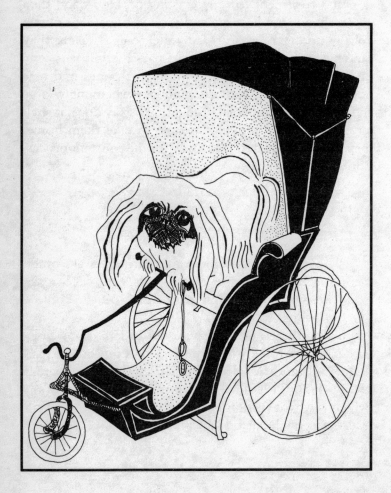

77. *Why am I always so tingly and itchy? My hair is dropping out in pawfuls.*

You're not alone. Itchiness is the most common reason that dogs visit veterinary clinics, and believe it or not fleas cause more itchiness than everything else combined.

Use a systematic approach to the problem. Look first for any sign of flea bites. Itchiness isn't caused by the fleas themselves but by the saliva they leave after sucking a meal. Although fleas are the most common cause of itchy skin disease, other skin parasites like ear mites, skin mites and lice can be equally or even more irritating.

Skin infection is also annoying. Fungal diseases, especially ringworm, can be quite irritating, while superficial or deep bacterial infections occur more frequently in certain breeds, such as cocker spaniels and golden retrievers, than in others.

Allergy to perfectly natural environmental components, such as grass or even to foods, causes itchy skin and, of course, plants like nettles that cause people to itch cause dogs to itch too.

Finally, there are more unusual causes. Poor blood circulation through the liver or interference in healthy kidney filtration can reveal themselves through tingly, itchy skin. Of course treatments vary dramatically, which is why it is so important to determine the specific cause of scratching and hair loss.

78. People are putting pills in my food to help me stop scratching but now I'm drinking like a fish. Are the pills making me thirsty?

Cortisone is the most effective anti-itch medicine for dogs and one of its most common side effects is a temporary increased thirst. Although this type of treatment is frequently absolutely necessary and marvellously effective when given for a short period of time, it can be more dangerous when used over prolonged periods.

Cortisone suppresses itch while the cause, parasites for example, is eliminated. It is not a cure. Sometimes the cause can't be eliminated. Some dogs, especially white or predominantly white-haired breeds, like West Highland white terriers and English setters, are allergic to dust mites, human dander, grass pollen or sap and other natural parts of the environment that in practical terms can't be eliminated. When this is the case and desensitising the dog is not possible, he needs medication to make life as pleasant as possible.

Antihistamines don't reduce itch in dogs as well as they do in people, but with recent improvements they should be tried. If one type has no effect in reducing scratching, another can be evaluated. Natural fats found in borage and evening primrose oil also reduce scratching but these need to be taken in large quantities, perhaps eight times the recommended dose; this can be quite expensive. Before embarking on this form of preventive treatment veterinary advice is very beneficial.

79. My bottom irritates me. I try to lick it and sometimes rub it on the grass and that h᷉ ᷉s. Do I have haemorrhoids?

Humans get haemorrhoids; dogs suffer from anal gland discomfort. They are similar only in that they are both irritating, although dogs can comfort and treat themselves in ways that people are not anatomically equipped to do.

Anal glands are part of the dog's territory-marking apparatus. After passing a stool, a dog squeezes anal gland discharge onto his droppings, marking them with his distinctive and unique scent. Some breeds, such as spaniels and dachshunds, have anatomically poorly placed glands that don't empty regularly. When they become full they irritate, so a dog empties them manually by licking or bum-dragging.

The discharge has a sharply distinctive smell that people find unpleasant. When anal glands become infected, instead of forming anal gland juice they fill with pus and even dogs find this fetid odour unpleasant. The discharge is sometimes blood-stained and dogs spend increasing parts of the day attending to their bottom. When this happens, the glands should be flushed out by the veterinarian with an antibiotic solution. Sometimes, when anal glands cause chronic irritation, they are surgically removed. To prevent infection from occurring, vets can show people how they can help dogs by squeezing empty the dog's scent sacs rather than relying upon the dog's licking and dragging to empty the irritating glands.

80. I am a happy, relaxed dog and have an interesting and varied life, but I can't control my intense desire to lick my forelegs whenever I lie down. Why do I behave so compulsively?

This is a unique form of skin complaint with no known physical cause. Happy-go-lucky Labradors and relaxed German shepherds are common indulgers in this form of compulsive behaviour.

Dogs who act this way only lick certain spots, almost invariably the last joint on the forelegs. When a dog is lying in his sphinx position, this is in fact the easiest spot to lick. He starts with a simple grooming lick but then keeps on licking. Sometimes he licks for so long he gets tired and falls asleep with his tongue extended in full licking position. After a few weeks of licking, the skin turns a mahogany colour, then hair disappears. The skin thickens and finally he breaks through to underlying tissue. Now the area tastes salty and far more interesting, so his licking becomes even more obsessive. Without any help from people, he will, if left on his own, lick right down to the bone.

Initially this is a psychological rather than a physical disease and is most similar to a human condition called obsessive compulsive disorder or OCD. People can try painting the licked area with something distasteful like bitter apple, but most dogs keep on licking. If medication is necessary, the problem often responds to the drugs used to treat OCD; in addition, the skin damage has to be repaired completely, otherwise when treatment stops they will go right back to licking again.

81. I enjoy sticking my dew claw in my ear, then licking the deliciously smelly wax I scrape onto it. What produces the wax and the smell?

The most likely cause is ear mites, although inhalation and dietary allergy also produce irritation and wax production, as do foreign bodies, such as grass seeds, in the ear canal. Ear mites or grass seeds or allergic reactions precipitate swelling and wax production, then bacteria, yeast and fungi move in. These are the smell producers, but they are secondary to the real cause.

Although dew claws are often removed from pups when they are a few days old, ear-digging is one purpose for which they are quite useful. The wax, mites, mite droppings and bacteria make a soupy stench that most dogs find attractive, but people find appalling.

Pups are most likely to have ear mites, a parting present from their mothers, but some breeds are always more prone to ear problems than others. Poodles, Yorkshire terriers, Lhasa Apsos and others with hair growing down the ear canals are predisposed to ear complaints because normal wax catches in the hair, providing an ideal environment in which bacteria can multiply. This is why hair should be plucked out of the ears routinely. Dramatically lop-eared breeds, especially those with heavily furred, pendulous flaps, like cocker spaniels, are prone to ear complaints because of poor air circulation and heightened humidity in the ear canal. Bugs thrive in hot climates. Routinely debulking the fur by shaving the inside of the ear flap reduces the likelihood of ear disease.

82. How can I explain to people that I have toothache?

When dogs drop food from their mouths, chew on one side or ask for but then don't eat food, they might have toothache. Pawing at the face and generally looking miserable are other possible signs. Most dogs are stoic about tooth pain and, because food is so important to them, gorge themselves as if nothing is wrong. The consequence is that suffering can go on for a considerable length of time before people notice.

Toothache is far more common than people realise. Because most dogs are inveterate chewers, there is a high risk that at some point during a dog's lifetime she will develop a hairline fracture or chip to a tooth. If this exposes the pulp, bacteria move into the root canal, producing an abscess. Often there are no outward signs of damage and these root abscesses only show up on dental X-rays.

Bad breath is a more obvious sign of gum disease, although it doesn't necessarily mean that pain is involved. The same applies to calculus on teeth. It might be unsightly and create a predisposition to infection, but its presence alone does not mean pain. Toothache can only be treated by getting to the root – if you'll pardon the term – of the problem. This usually means removing the offending tooth, although there is no reason why a tooth should not be saved by having a root canal filling. Many veterinarians have both the equipment and the experience to carry out this dental procedure.

83. When I looked recently I noticed I have only one testicle. Should I be concerned?

It is too late to be concerned. Dogs with only one testicle are useless for show purposes, although some dogs have had silicone testicle implants. Their fertility is only moderately lower than normal, so a retained testicle does not prevent successful breeding. The problem is genetic, and much more common in some breeds than in others, so sex is best avoided if the problem is to be controlled.

It should be controlled because there is a much higher incidence of cancer in retained testicles than in fully descended ones. Testicles are built to be most efficient at a temperature a few degrees lower than inside the body. That is why they migrated out of the abdominal cavity in the first place. Retained testicles find themselves in a hotter environment, which is why the sperm produced by them are not as healthy and also why tumours are more likely to develop.

If a dog has one or both testicles retained, he should have a complete physical examination each year. Sometimes the retained testicles are in the inguinal canal between the abdomen and the scrotum and are easy to feel. At other times they remain nestled up near the kidneys, where they began life. At the very first sign of any possible increase in size they should be surgically removed.

84. Are so-called alternative forms of medicine like homeopathy and acupuncture just for people or can I derive benefit from them too?

Alternative medicine is for dogs too, but don't expect frequent miracles. These are safe and perhaps even sensible and beneficial treatments for chronic conditions. But when there is an acute problem, a serious infection for example, it is quite irresponsible to rely on the unknown value of an alternative form of medicine when conventional medicine – a course of antibiotics in the case of an infection – will produce a cure.

Alternative medicine is most appropriate when conventional medicine fails. Acupuncture, whatever its mechanism of action, might help to reduce pain when other methods have failed. Herbal medicines are without doubt beneficial for treating numerous conditions. After all, willow bark was chewed to reduce pain by North American Indians for hundreds of years before aspirin was derived from it. Homeopathic treatments, such as arnica and hypericum, will certainly cause no harm and may be beneficial to prevent or to treat bruising and tissue damage.

Good nursing is one of the most important factors in treating any medical condition in people or in dogs. A great advantage of alternative forms of medicine is that they are almost invariably given with great enthusiasm. And when treatments are carried out this way, it doesn't matter whether the patient is a biped or quadruped, he knows he is loved and wanted. That alone will help him to get better faster.

85. Recently and quite suddenly I have been leaving small floods and piles in the house at night. Is this a normal result of advancing age or is it the first sign of canine Alzheimer's?

Alzheimer's has never been diagnosed in dogs, although it is likely to occur. Incontinence is a sign of illness or a natural consequence of aging and loss of control of the right muscles.

There are possible medical reasons for urinary incontinence. Bladder infection irritates the lining of the urinary system, making dribbling more likely. And some females, especially Dobermanns, springer spaniels and Old English sheepdogs, become incontinent after they are spayed because of associated hormone changes and the fact that their bladders are not in the best position in the first place. Either hormone supplements or surgery, or both, will correct the problem.

Double incontinence, involving both the bladder and bowels, almost always means poor muscle tone. This can be a sign of generalised illness, but when it occurs in otherwise healthy pensioners, anabolic steroids, the nasties that athletes abuse, can sometimes improve old age loss of muscle control. Diet changes help too. Sometimes sex hormones work wonders. Whatever the cause, people should remember that it is unfair to discipline a dog for doing something she has no control over. Many dogs are just as upset over their loss of sanitary habits as people are.

86. How can I explain to people that my not answering when they call my name is not because I'm becoming stubborn but because I'm going deaf?

Deafness is difficult for people to recognise, especially in older dogs, because they can't decide whether a lack of response is caused by increasing independence or hearing loss.

Deafness is unusual in young dogs and occurs frequently only in certain predominantly white breeds, especially varieties of bull terrier, Dalmatians and Sealyhams. These dogs are born hearing but go deaf by the time they are twelve weeks old. It is a hereditary form of deafness, and the risk will be passed on if the deaf dog breeds.

Masses of ear wax will certainly reduce hearing, although on its own this doesn't cause deafness. Needless to say, routinely cleaning the ears controls this cause of hearing impairment.

As age-related hearing loss occurs – and this is very common in golden retrievers over twelve – dogs compensate for their loss by using their other senses more acutely. They know people are approaching them by feeling the vibrations of human footsteps in the floor. How they know the fridge has been opened several floors away remains a mystery, however. Hearing loss is just as natural in dogs as it is in people; old age wear and tear is the most likely cause. Dogs can best communicate their hearing loss by failing to respond to quietly spoken joy words like 'food', 'park', 'eat' and 'walk'.

87. I don't understand why my legs hurt when I first get up in the morning but feel better after I have had exercise.

This is caused by a gradual loss of lubricating fluids in the joints, with associated mild but chronic joint inflammation or arthritis.

Large breeds are more prone to morning lameness than others. Many breeds, such as German shepherds and Labrador retrievers, have a high incidence of inherited hip joint arthritis or dysplasia. While they are young and their muscles are fit and well toned this arthritis causes no problem but with aging lameness occurs. Other breeds, such as Rottweilers and Pyrenean mountain dogs, are often born with shoulder joint problems called OC. The milder the problem, the less likely it is that it will cause lameness while a dog is young, but the joint will hurt later on in life.

These joints hurt most after they have been rested, which is why lameness is worst when a dog first moves. After a little exercise the muscles get worked in and discomfort diminishes. These dogs should never have sudden excessive exercise, for that will exaggerate the lameness. They thrive on routine daily exercise and respond to non-steroid anti-inflammatories like aspirin, which is sometimes given preventively as well as therapeutically.

88. I think I need glasses. Things aren't as clear as they used to be and my eyes are getting cloudy. Am I getting cataracts?

Compared with people all dogs have poor vision close up and would benefit from glasses. The idea is, of course, impractical, although contact lenses have been developed and artificial lenses have been implanted in dogs' eyes to restore vision.

Dogs have excellent distance vision, but as they mature their lenses lose their ability to focus accurately. That is why older dogs have difficulty seeing people or objects right in front of their eyes, although they still see distant moving objects quite clearly. Over the years the lenses themselves start to lose their clarity, and after ten years a cloudiness develops. Light entering the eyes has to pass through these foggy lenses and some of this light reflects back, making the eyes appear blue-grey. This is a normal aging change.

Cataracts are quite different. Outwardly cataracts appear similar to the cloudiness of natural age change. But, in fact, impenetrable crystals form in the lenses, preventing images from passing through to be seen by the retina. This causes blindness. Cataract-damaged lenses can be surgically removed and, in some instances, replaced by artificial lenses, but only if the retina is in fine working condition. Many cataracts are hereditary in nature and are accompanied by hereditary deterioration to the retina called progressive retinal atrophy or PRA. When PRA accompanies cataracts, surgery, unfortunately, is almost always pointless.

89. Although I look and feel fine, over the last month I've become thirstier and thirstier. Is it just the weather or could it be anything serious?

A prolonged increased thirst almost always means that something potentially serious is happening. Weather alone won't dramatically increase water consumption.

Poor kidney function is the most common reason why older dogs drink more, although kidney problems and associated thirst can also occur as a hereditary disease in certain breeds, such as cocker spaniels, when they are less than two years old. Kidney function is tested rapidly by checking a blood sample for levels of waste products. If a blood test reveals that the kidneys are having problems, then protein in the diet – meat – should be drastically reduced.

Bladder infection, liver problems, sugar diabetes and other diseases such as adrenal and pituitary gland disorders all stimulate thirst. These, too, can be diagnosed through tests on blood samples, urine samples, or both, but they require medical management rather than simple dietary changes. Treatments for other conditions, such as cortisone for itchy skin, also create thirst. A final curious reason for excessive drinking is strictly psychological. When some dogs get overexcited, they compulsively drink copious quantities of water. This can happen at unexpected times, when a dog comes *back* from kennels for example. He drinks like a camel for several days and then quite spontaneously reverts back to his natural consumption. No treatment is necessary because the problem is self-limiting.

90. People have arranged to leave me at the veterinarian's for an operation. Aren't anaesthetics dangerous and isn't surgery painful?

There is a statistical danger associated with anaesthetics, and surgery is just as painful for dogs as it is for people, but both of these potential worries can be reduced through care and common sense.

Dogs should fast before having anaesthetics administered. This eliminates the possibility that they will vomit while they are asleep. They should also submit to complete physical examinations, especially of their heart and lungs. Sometimes, if there are any reasons for concern, blood tests should be carried out before an anaesthetic to make sure that liver and kidney function are normal. If there are any abnormalities, then the method of anaesthesia can be modified to compensate.

Many anaesthetics act as mild pain killers but all surgery is potentially painful, especially surgery inside body cavities and on bones. Pain killers should be liberally given, not just when dogs say they are in pain – many dogs are too stoic to let on they are suffering – but routinely before, during and after surgery. Most dogs are far better than people at recovering from surgery. They don't have abstract psychological problems, which is why they improve so rapidly. It is important not to kill pain completely, however. Pain is the body's way of telling itself to take it easy. A little mild discomfort after surgery is not a bad thing, for it keeps the patients still and prevents post-surgical complications.

CHAPTER EIGHT

Grooming and Preventive Care

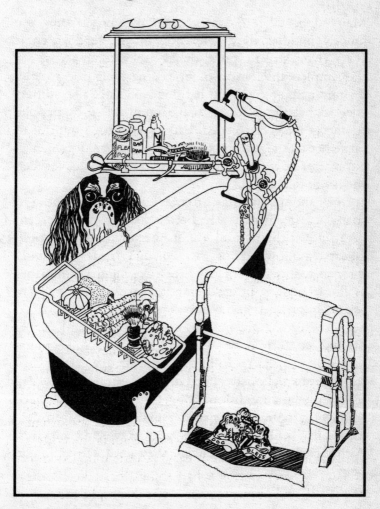

91. I like water on my own terms, not when people throw it on me. How often should I bathe and groom?

Many dogs take to water naturally. When they see muddy puddles they belly flop in. These dogs enter every river, stream, pond or lake they come across for the simple exhilaration of practising their dog paddle. Swimming is enjoyed but bathing is endured. The difference is that the latter is forced upon a dog by people. As far as she is concerned, bathing is carried out not to make her clean but as a simple act of human dominance. No matter how much she likes water, she hates it when she is not in control.

Dogs should swim as often as they like but bathe in soapy water infrequently because soap and detergent break down the natural oils in the fur. Bathing should be carried out when dogs stink or their fur is sufficiently dirty to require it. The need for soapy baths diminishes as the frequency of grooming increases. Dogs who are routinely brushed and combed rarely need to be bathed because regular grooming keeps the skin and fur in pristine condition. Some dogs, like birds, give themselves dust baths by rolling in sand or dry earth. This, too, is a marvellously effective and natural way to keep hair in the best condition. Long, thin coated breeds need frequent grooming to prevent matts of hair forming, especially behind their ears and between their legs. Although licking is beneficial, they need active human help to groom effectively.

92. Should I use any special shampoo to eliminate body odour?

Dogs should use shampoos and conditioners that are most appropriate for the texture, density and length of their coats. For example, a wire-haired fox terrier should avoid conditioners if he wants to live up to his name, while a silky terrier should always use one after each and every shampoo.

If a dog is healthy and fit, he should not suffer from body odour. Routine brushing and combing prevents most smell. If he does smell strongly, there is usually a specific reason, for example an ear infection or, if he is a spaniel, a lip fold infection, and these should be treated appropriately.

General body odour can be related to diet, but dog smell is also exaggerated when the oil-producing glands that keep his hair shiny and waterproof go into over-production. When this happens his coat becomes oily or dandruffy and he should use an anti-dandruff shampoo. Selenium, coal tar and benzoyl peroxide shampoos are all used, but zinc pyrithion, which people often apply for dandruff, might be dangerous if used frequently. As an alternative to conditioners, dogs can use products called humectants on their coats. These increase the suppleness of their skin and reduce dandruff without making their hair oily. They can be used as frequently as is necessary.

93. Be honest, is there really anything terribly wrong with me biting my own nails?

There is nothing wrong with nail biting as long as a dog doesn't bite off so much that he makes his nails bleed; in fact, people are far more likely to do that. Medium and large sized dogs wear down their nails naturally and have no need to bite them until they are older and their nails grow longer. On the other hand, very small canines weigh so little that without frequent nail grooming theirs grow excessively long and interfere with walking and running.

A typical nail biter simply lies down and munches at his claws, biting off the sharp tips. Some munchers lie on their backs, using one paw to hold down the other for grooming. Most dogs, however, need human help with this procedure.

All pups should have their nails cut when they are between eight and twelve weeks old. Only the sharp point of the nail is cut off. This is best done with a nail clipper that uses a guillotine action. Clippers that crush, scissor-like, between two blades can cause pain if nails are thick, as they will be later in life.

Inside the nail there is living tissue and this is what bleeds and hurts when it is accidentally severed. It can be seen and avoided in pearly lustred white nails, but is invisible within dark nails. All weight-bearing nails get routine wear, but dew claws have little activity or function, so these need most attention, especially in breeds such as the Pekingese where they frequently grow back around on themselves and can puncture the skin. All nails should be inspected and groomed monthly.

94. Why won't people let me exercise? They say they won't let me off my lead until I grow up.

People often worry needlessly that a pup will damage himself if he has too much exercise while he is young. As long as his activity is not extreme, there is no reason why he shouldn't be let off his lead so that he can indulge in typical puppy mayhem. Wolf cubs do this and they come to no harm as a result.

There is one mild exception and that applies to the giant, fast-growing breeds such as St Bernards and Great Danes. These breeds grow unnaturally quickly. Many people wrongly feel that these dogs should have no exercise off a lead until they are physically mature. This is not so. Their rapid rate of growth does predispose them to bone development problems, but denying them exercise is not the answer. These dogs need well-balanced diets with neither too little nor too much calcium and phosphorus. Meat is high in phosphorus and low in calcium. Phosphorus prevents calcium from getting to bones where it is needed, so high phosphorus diets are harmful to all dogs but especially to fast-growing ones. A diet consisting of slightly more calcium than phosphorus, with Vitamin D, allows for good bone development. As long as a pup is well nourished, even giant breed pups can be allowed off their leads each day to have moderate controlled exercise.

95. I've got worms and they make my bottom itchy. How did I get them and how can I get rid of them?

Tapeworm segments cause bottom itch because they crawl in and out, producing irritation. A dog's other worms – roundworms, hookworms and whipworms – usually stay further inside where they can cause considerable damage but no itchiness.

To provide a home for a tapeworm a dog must consume a tapeworm egg. This is most commonly done by eating a flea that already contains the egg. Uncooked fish can be a source of another tapeworm; offal from sheep, goats, pigs, cattle, or even kangaroo for that matter, is yet another source of tapeworm eggs. In the intestines, an egg matures into an adult worm which, if it is the common flea-transmitted tapeworm, then releases egg-filled segments which meander out of the dog's bottom. Once in the outside world these eggs are eaten by flea larvae, the larvae mature into adult fleas, which the dog accidentally eats while grooming himself, and the tapeworm life-cycle has been completed.

Roundworms, hookworms and whipworms either are picked up from the environment or are a gift to pups from their mother before they are born. They seldom cause anal irritation but are sometimes vomited or passed in the dog's stool. All of these worms can be virtually eliminated by routine worming and defleaing. Pregnant females should be wormed frequently before birth, pups wormed several times while still only a few weeks old and all dogs at least twice yearly.

96. Where do all those creepers that enjoy living on and in my skin come from?

Mites, lice and fleas come from other animals, not necessarily just from other dogs. The very young, the elderly and the debilitated are those most likely to have these fellow travellers.

Demodex mites are contracted by pups from their mothers just after birth and are present in the hair follicles of many healthy dogs, but in short-haired breeds such as Dobermanns and bull terriers they sometimes multiply excessively and cause serious skin disease. A deficiency in a dog's immune system is probably what allows them to multiply, which is why routine anti-parasite shampoos are not very effective in controlling them. More potent treatments are needed.

Scabies mites are contracted from other infected animals, including other dogs. Foxes are a common source (in Australia so are wombats), and as foxes become more urban, the incidence of scabies in dogs increases. These mites burrow deeply in the skin, which is why insecticidal shampoos must be applied for several consecutive weeks.

Biting and sucking lice are also maternal gifts. They are a sign of poor hygiene; they live on the skin surface and glue their tiny shiny eggs to hair. These are readily eliminated, as are fleas, with an insecticidal shampoo or spray.

97. How can I best control my terror and panic when I visit the veterinary clinic?

First impressions can last forever and it is unfortunate that the first time a dog visits a veterinary clinic he gets stabbed in the back. This is an unavoidable unpleasantry, so his visit should in all other ways be made as enjoyable as possible.

Very often he is already frightened because he has just had his first car ride, he is with people he doesn't know and he hears other animal noises that signal distress or danger. In the best of all possible circumstances, the veterinary clinic should provide a clean area where the pup can be put down, if only to find his feet again. He will probably want to empty his bladder, and if at the same time he comes across a treat to sniff and eat, his first impression will be a positive one.

People often transmit their own fear of visiting the doctor or dentist or veterinarian to their dog. Even young pups are exquisitely sensitive to people's behaviour. Dog owners often worry needlessly that the vet will tell them their new pup is a dud, is riddled with parasites, has four left feet or is a rat in disguise. They worry that the pup will be frightened or experience pain. The young pup picks up the owner's feelings of apprehension and he gets nervous. People should act as relaxed as possible when taking a dog to the veterinary clinic.

Once he is on the examining table, the dog should be approached at his own level. He should be allowed to walk over to his examiner and carry out an investigation.

When this has been completed, the examiner can investigate him. Injections are more painful to some dogs than to others. Breeds such as Labradors seldom notice that anything has happened, while Cavalier King Charles spaniels shriek as if the end of the world has come. As most dogs can't concentrate on two things at once, now is a good time for another food treat to be offered. An injection is given while the pup investigates or eats the food he has just discovered. If this first trip is turned into an enjoyable occasion, it will make future visits easier. At home people can open a dog's mouth, look in his ears, part his hair, lift his tail and in other ways examine him as the vet does. This is ultimately of importance because easy dogs get more complete medical examinations and that makes diagnoses faster and better.

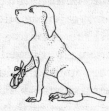

98. I've never met a dog that has had distemper. Is vaccination really worth the pain?

Yes, it is. Twenty years ago distemper was a relatively common disease. It is only because of effective vaccination programmes that it is now so uncommon in many parts of the world. Where routine vaccination is not carried out distemper is still a frequent cause of illness and death.

The value of routine vaccination against rabies where that virus exists is obvious. Inoculation protects both dogs and humans. But there are many other diseases both local or national against which dogs can be protected. Leptospirosis is spread through rat urine. It kills people and dogs each year but prevention is simple through vaccination. Parvovirus didn't exist in dogs until the late 1970s, when it suddenly spread around the world, wiping out complete litters overnight. This is easily controlled through vaccination as well. So, too, are virus hepatitis and causes of less important but still troublesome kennel cough. Protection against all of these diseases is incorporated into a single vaccine. If there are specific diseases that occur in certain regions, risk of contracting them can also be reduced through vaccination. Lyme disease spread by ticks, Bordatella, a whooping cough-like kennel cough and other infections that occur either seasonally or regionally can be prevented through routine vaccination. It all boils down to an argument over which is preferable, prevention or cure. Today sensible dogs and people opt for the former.

99. Sometimes my nose is wet; at other times it is dry. Does it matter?

It doesn't matter one tiny bit. The state of the nose depends upon what a dog is doing or has recently been doing, as well as the type of climate.

Sleeping dogs frequently have dry noses; upon awakening they usually stretch their bodies and then lick their proboscises. A wet nose is useful because scent molecules are trapped in the moisture and can be inhaled either into the nasal chambers themselves or up into the vomeronasal organ where sex scent is analysed. When dogs are exercising, their noses are usually wet because exercise is the pet dog's equivalent of hunting; scenting ability should be at its best then.

Dogs can't sweat the way people do and in warm weather wearing fur can be oppressive. Heavy panting eliminates excess heat and moisture and here, too, the nose can be moderately useful. Moisture evaporates off a wet nose, but the appendage may be hot or cold depending upon the surrounding temperature. The same applies indoors. The only circumstance in which the state of the nose is important is when dogs have fevers. A cold wet nose usually means there is no fever. A hot wet nose can be normal or can indicate that body temperature is above normal. It is only of significance when dogs show other signs of illness.

100. I hate taking medicine. What is the least distasteful way of doing so?

Receiving medicine by injection is the most reliable way and, curiously, often the least distasteful. Sometimes, as when treating sugar diabetes, it is the only way that medicine can be taken. Insulin injections are given with a very thin needle under the skin on the neck, one of the least sensitive parts of the body. Because it is part of the daily routine and is relatively innocuous, most dogs don't mind.

Many people have a deep aversion to needles. They don't like receiving medicine from them and hate the thought of giving medicine with them. That's why most drugs are in liquid, capsule or tablet form. Human preferences do not necessarily apply to canines. Some dogs think that taking medicine by mouth is the most horrific torture devised by humans. They clamp their jaws shut, refusing to open the necessary orifice or, if they do open up, they try to clamp down on the fingers giving the medicine.

Liquids can be more difficult to consume, especially if they are ladled into a dog's mouth with a spoon. Plastic syringes are useful as administrators. The syringe is filled with the liquid which is then gently squirted into the dog's mouth with care that none gets down the windpipe.

Capsules and pills can be more difficult. Small dogs, in particular, seem to have unexplored hidden recesses deep in their mouth cavities in which they can hide pills for hours before spitting them out. Special plastic pill pushers can be used but these are potentially dangerous. It is preferable to hide the medicine. Cubes of meat work wonders, as does Cheddar cheese, although some antibiotics should not be given with dairy products. If a dog refuses to eat and must have his medicine, there is no alternative for a human but to hold his mouth open towards the sky and to drop the offensive object as far down as possible. The mouth should be clamped shut and the neck rubbed. Dry pills can be greased with vegetable oil. Alternatively, a few drops of water can be squirted into the clamped-shut mouth. A nose lick means the medicine has gone down. Because dogs should always 'come' on command, people should never call them for such unpleasant indignities as pill-giving.

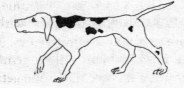

101. Is there life after death?

You need a theologian rather than a veterinarian to answer that question. There is a unique difference between many human deaths and dog deaths in that active euthanasia is rare in the former but common with the latter. Because so many dogs are living for so long, people increasingly are forced to make life and death decisions about when a dog should die.

Death itself is very peaceful. A dog is simply given an anaesthetic and falls asleep. While he is asleep, his heart stops. Then, depending upon where he has lived and what people want, he is usually either cremated or buried.

In countries with Judaeo-Christian traditions some people feel there is an afterlife for themselves but not for their dogs. In one survey one in five felt that dogs have an afterlife, while over twice as many felt that they themselves would have life after death. There are different attitudes elsewhere. In Japan surveys show equal numbers of people feel that dogs and people have souls and afterlives. The dog's cardinal advantage over humans is that throughout his life he doesn't think about an afterlife. He approaches the end of his natural existence with dignity and dies without needing answers. Many humans who believe in an afterlife, however, hope that when they finally get there, dogs will be waiting.

List of Questions

119

CHAPTER TWO   Emotions and Behaviour

CHAPTER THREE **Training**

CHAPTER SEVEN   Illness and Disease

CHAPTER EIGHT   Grooming and Preventive Care

Index